# The Eight Human Talents

# The Eight Human Talents

## Restore the Balance and Serenity within You with Kundalini Yoga

### Gurmukh Kaur Khalsa
with Cathryn Michon

HARPER

NEW YORK · LONDON · TORONTO · SYDNEY

The material contained within this book is informational only. It is not intended to diagnose, treat, cure, or be a substitute for medical supervision. Please consult your physician for treatment of all medical conditions.

The poem "A Blessing for the Senses" from *Anam Cara: A Book of Celtic Wisdom* by John O'Donohue is reprinted by permission of HarperCollins Publishers Inc. Copyright ©1997 by John O'Donohue.

HarperCollins books may be purchased for educational, business, or sales promotional use. For information, please e-mail the Special Markets Department at SPsales@harpercollins.com.

First Cliff Street Books paperback edition published 2001

*Designed by Jeannette Jacobs*
*Illustrations by Pearl Beach*

Library of Congress Cataloging-in-Publication Data has been applied for.

ISBN 0-06-019548-7
ISBN 0-06-095465-5 (pbk.)

16 17 ❖/RRD 30 29 28 27 26 25 24 23 22

## A PRAYER FOR YOU

Let the wind be behind you,

Angels dance with you

And your consciousness

Guide you to victory.

Let the Angels,

The Great Souls, the Avatars,

And all Incarnations of God

Pray for you.

Walk tall and bless all,

In your innocence with your love,

For each one's peace

And prosperity.

Remember what time wants;

Serve the needs of the time and space.

You will be sacred, exalted,

Beautiful, bountiful and fulfilled.

—*Yogi Bhajan*

This book is dedicated to my beloved teacher, Yogi Bhajan, and the Golden Chain of Teachers before him who together brought these ancient teachings to the West, to us, the wanderers of the sixties; to my parents, who gave me life; and to my dear daughter, Wahe Guru Kaur, her entire generation, and the five generations to follow; to all the students who have passed through our doors during these last thirty years, having been transformed as a result of these teachings; and to all those who are now teaching Kundalini Yoga and Meditation throughout the world.

# CONTENTS

# FOREWORD

In this changing world, humans are being eaten inside by deep depression. It is an urgent need of the time to reverse this process. There are zillions of thoughts, millions of feelings, hundreds of thousands of emotions, and thousands of desires. This is the grinding wheel through which humanity is being milled, and we have to reverse this grinding wheel of pain into a force of happiness—happiness which is our birthright. This work serves that purpose. May God bless all those who practice this.

—*Yogi Bhajan*

# INDEX OF EXERCISES AND DIAGRAMS

# ACKNOWLEDGMENTS

I wish to thank my dear editor at HarperCollins, Diane Reverand; Jane Dystel and her agency for her confidence in the work; Cathryn Michon, who had the vision; Tej Kaur, who took the project to the end; my husband, Gurushabd Singh, who keeps me grounded; Marlene Stevens, who has been right by my side in support and love; and all the students at Golden Bridge who cheered me on.

# A Personal Glimpse

Let me introduce myself to those who don't yet know me. My name is Gurmukh, and I have had the great blessing to be a teacher of Kundalini Yoga for almost thirty years. Kundalini Yoga is a beautiful and ancient science, which was once held highly guarded and very secret. This yoga has the potential to heal and uplift anyone's life for the better.

I first met my beloved spiritual teacher, Yogi Bhajan, in 1971, in Tucson, Arizona. As the Master of Kundalini Yoga, his mission has been to create teachers of this sacred science since his arrival in the United States in 1969. I was in awe when I first laid eyes on him. I quietly presented myself before him, and he looked at me with his penetrating gaze. He gave me my name, "Gurmukh," right there at our first meeting—a name which literally means one who lives and breathes words of divine wisdom and communicates that essence deeply from her heart.

I also remember what he told me at that time. "You don't know what would have happened to you if you hadn't come to this path. You would have gone through so much. You will be totally transformed."

It is with deep gratitude for the experience of my soul that I have dedicated my life to helping others find their own soul-connection through the vehicle of Kundalini Yoga and Meditation. I don't believe this to be the only way to dive into our inner depths, but I have seen how quickly and powerfully it changes people from a state of misery to that of serenity, and even ecstasy.

I live with my husband and daughter in Los Angeles. We recently opened a beautiful yoga center here called "Golden Bridge." I am grateful this center helps and serves as a sanctuary for so many.

I am a Sikh. Every year I go to India to renew my spirit, letting her teach me and bend me as she will. I have learned many of my greatest spiritual lessons in that strange and beautiful land.

We go many places in India, but mostly north to the the Golden Temple in Amritsar, the spiritual home of the Sikhs. This magnificent golden building, where prayer and chanting have been continuous for more than four hundred years, is surrounded by a big body of water. There are vortexes on the earth that have a high frequency and are said to hold the world together. In these places, people are continuously praying for peace on earth. The Golden Temple, with its four doors open to people of all walks of life, is one of these places.

At the Golden Temple, ten thousand people are fed every day, and housing is provided. When people pray, sing, and eat together, there will be peace on earth.

My next great love in India is Dharamsala, where His Holiness, the Dalai Lama, lives among the exiled Tibetan Buddhists. Theirs is such a gentle culture. When you see the bumper stickers on cars in America, "Free Tibet," they are saying, "Save the tradition of compassion."

On my most recent trip, God gave me a gift I will never forget. I was walking down the town's main dirt road. I turned the corner and saw people gathered on either side of the road. There were nuns, monks, Tibetan children, the shopkeepers, so many people. It was quite a festive gathering. The Indians were selling popcorn, and everyone in town seemed to be there.

They were waiting for the Dalai Lama's motorcade to pass through. He was coming up from the temple and his home to go to Delhi, where he was to fly to Israel and then on to Africa. We waited all together. Little village puppies were running around. Security was trying to keep the road clear. I was tightly tucked between a nun and monk. Across the way, the kids were playing. A train of donkeys carried granite to the temple. Foreigners were scattered in the crowd. Every time a car approached, we thought it was he.

The moment finally arrived. From the bottom of the hill came the golden-colored car, with security jeeps in front and back, moving slowly. As his car approached us, I caught a glimpse of His Holiness with his hands in a prayer at his forehead, bowing with a smile.

Then something happened. Time stood still. Everything merged: colors blended, nothing moved. As his car swept by, I heard a hushed sound of "Ahh"—a sound that resounded from the very core of all who were present, and for that brief moment everything became One. I was awed at that moment by the warmth and radiance that can emanate from one great soul. The radiance of this holy man completely overtook us all.

There have been only a few times in my life that I have experienced this wonderful feeling of oneness. It was the same feeling as when my daughter came forth into this world. The oneness I felt in Dharamsala that day lasted only a moment. The Dalai Lama drove off, up the road, and disappeared. The colors separated, time started moving, and we were back—but somehow we were all a little altered. This humble man gave us the *experience* of the human radiance, developed to its fullest.

It will be my great privilege and honor if this book can be an inspiration, and if even only on a small level, causes its own ripple effect to bring a little more joy and expansion into the lives of others. Sat Nam.

—*Gurmukh Kaur Khalsa*

# INTRODUCTION

One day someone asked me what I used to be like before I did Kundalini Yoga and Meditation. I stared a moment, not out of rudeness, but because I honestly cannot remember. I am a very different person now. I believe that in doing this work, following the way of yoga and meditation, I have healed and blossomed on a cellular level, and connected with the truth of my soul's journey. In so doing, I have also been of service to others. All this has happened in my life because of this incredibly profound healing technology called Kundalini Yoga and Meditation. I believe that part of my purpose here in this lifetime is to bring what I have learned to others.

I am so enthusiastic about the miracles I have seen happen with yoga and meditation. **Learning to meditate will attract all that you are longing to understand.**

**It's not the life that you live, it's the courage that you bring to it.**

When the challenges in life come, as they do to everyone, I have tools I use to begin healing myself. Some of them are very simple and take only a few minutes of my time.

**Yoga is not about self-improvement, it's about self-acceptance.**

More and more, people are becoming drawn to yoga and meditation, and this does not surprise me at all. It's important to understand doing yoga is not just another "self-improvement" craze. Yoga is not a practice of self-improvement at all. It is a practice of *self-acceptance*, which is a very different thing. You don't need to be "fixed"; you simply need to reconnect with how wonderful and perfect you already are. Yoga is about remembering who you truly are. That is why doing yoga, even on the smallest level, can change the course of your life, just as it has mine. Your birthright is happiness. You are born as a spiritual being to have a human experience.

In Kundalini Yoga, the biggest challenge is usually not the exercise itself, it is getting myself just to do it! The fact that I teach yoga for a living doesn't mean that I always remember to use it when I most need it. Sometimes I know that I need to refocus and that it's worth taking three or five minutes to do something to make myself feel better, and yet my negative mind will still win the battle. Sometimes getting myself just to do it is harder than any super-advanced yoga handstand I could try.

**Misery is a choice we can count on. Misery is not elusive, it's always there for us.**

If we can make one step towards happiness, towards healing, towards change, miracles begin to happen. The Kundalini Yoga and Meditation in this book are a way of making those small steps towards happiness.

If you will try even one thing from this book—one breathing exercise, one stretch, one meditation—know that somewhere I am cheering right out loud for you, because I know making that first step is the hardest thing to do, and in just doing it, even once, you have achieved an enormous victory for yourself!

## Mantras: How They Work

In Kundalini Yoga, we often accompany a movement or even a breath pattern with sounds we sing or meditate on silently, called "mantras."

Mantras are repetitive sounds we make over and over to bring about a change in our consciousness.

Chanting may seem strange to you at first, but it is a powerful tool for healing. People often ask me what is the purpose of a certain chant in a certain meditation. The words are chosen not only for their meaning as words, but also for a scientific reason that goes far beyond pure definition. All mantras we use are based on the science of "Naad"—the secrets hidden in sound.

The roof of our mouth has eighty-four meridian points, all along the upper palate. Mantras were given to us as special gifts. Long ago, highly evolved beings went into deeply meditative states. They began reciting certain sounds that made the tongue hit these meridian points in the mouth in certain combinations. It's kind of like playing the piano—if certain notes are struck, a beautiful song is produced. With every word we speak, or in this case the mantras we recite, we hit certain "keys." If the right combination of keys is struck, then the hypothalamus, thalamus, and pituitary in the brain are all stimulated in such a way as to bring our minds into a meditative state, and even into ecstasy. And just think, if we can produce that state without drugs, what a world this would be.

This is also why sometimes you'll walk into a room in which people have been gossiping, swearing a lot, or generally talking "low-vibrational" talk, and the whole room will feel depressed and heavy. Other times, you might walk into a room in which a lot of chanting or uplifting kinds of conversations have been occurring, and you'll feel a lightness and ease in the room. What you're experiencing has a lot to do with the science of Naad.

Each mantra was chosen by those ancient wise people because it encapsulated an uplifting vibration into a few choice little words. When we recite them, we stimulate certain parts of our brain that actually change the chemical balance of the brain. This changed chemical composition allows a more relaxed and expanded state of consciousness to overtake our minds.

**"In the coming age, the mental insanity, which has started breeding now and which will multiply and multiply, will not**

be curable by any medicine. At that moment the practice of chanting in Naad yoga will be most effective.

It will bring about a balanced state of mind."

—Yogi Bhajan

One of the most powerful mantras we use in Kundalini yoga is "Sat Nam," meaning "I am Truth." The beautiful pure vowel sounds are very similar to the Latin "Amen." We end each yoga class with a long, sung "Sat Nam."

We all use mantras all day long—repetitive, out loud, or silently—phrases such as "It's hard," or "I'm tired." "I don't know what I'm doing," "It will never happen," "I'm stressed," "There's not enough time," or "There's not enough money."

We don't even notice them becoming part of our reality by repetition. We act out on what we say, live on how we think. If your mantra is, "I am stressed," you will be stressed. Or if your mantra is, "It's never going to happen,"—it's never going to happen. In the beginning was the word, and the word was God. So powerful are our words to ourselves and to others.

## MUDRAS: MAGIC HAND POSITIONS

Along with the use of mantras, we sometimes use "mudras" in Kundalini Yoga and Meditation. These special hand positions are designed to bring energies into the body, and along with the use of mantras and eye focal points, they send certain messages to our brain. They aid in producing calming and meditative states within our being.

## CHAKRAS

The purpose of this book is to provide you with small ways to help you become aware of your own chakra centers, and enrich your life by tapping into the vast technology of Kundalini Yoga and Meditation.

"Men of great knowledge actually found out about all these chakras—their workings, their petals, their sounds, their infinity, their co-relationship, their powers. They found out what the chakras were. And, they found out that the life of a human is totally based on these chakras. They developed it into a whole science. This total science gave birth to Kundalini Yoga. That is how Kundalini Yoga was born."

—Yogi Bhajan

Chakra is the Sanskrit word for "wheel." Think of your chakras as spinning vortexes, each radiating a particular energy that's important to your health, happiness, and well-being. These eight energy centers begin at the base of your spine and continue upward to the top of your head, as shown in the illustration at the end of this chapter.

"The energy of the universe is yours. It is your birthright. Just claim it."

—Yogi Bhajan

These centers are divided into the "lower triangle," which refers to the first three chakras, and the "upper triangle." They meet in the middle at the navel point. The eighth chakra, the aura, is like a bubble surrounding the entire physical structure, and is a culmination or reflection of the being as a whole.

Chakras are complex, radiating more than one quality or emotion. To help you begin to understand how they operate, I have distilled each chakra to one human talent and one shadow emotion in this book.

The Eight Human Talents are those gifts that make human beings different from every other animal on earth.

"Talent will take you everywhere. There is nothing which talent cannot create. There is nowhere that talent cannot reach. It will give you every spot. It will give you every place.

Talent is the vehicle of Infinity, which is yours in which you
use your consciousness and intuition."

—Yogi Bhajan

Each chakra is associated with a particular talent, gift, or skill we
can gain to enhance our lives, when the chakra is open and vibrating at
maximum intensity. Each is traditionally associated with a particular
color.

Sometimes people will refer to a negative emotional state, a psychological difficulty, associated with a particular chakra. These are not necessarily "set in stone" associations, since emotions tend to overlap and
intermix with each other. To simplify, I have linked the chakras to
"shadow emotions," if you will, and have described yogic tools to help a
person deal with the darker side of the human psyche.

"Don't solve your problems, dissolve your problems—so they
should not reoccur again."

—Yogi Bhajan

These wonderful chakras make humans different from every other
animal on earth. When we begin to honor the power and develop the talents they offer, we will heal as individuals and as a species.

My teacher, Yogi Bhajan, taught me to think of chakras as gears of a car.
Each is important and useful for getting where you want to go. We call Kundalini Yoga the "Yoga of Awareness," because it teaches you how to become
aware of the energies you contain, and then teaches you how to "shift gears"
smoothly when you need to.

"To be successful in life, you have to learn to change your
gears to meet the circumstances around you. If you are not in
control of your own transmission, life will be a disaster for
you, no matter who you are. You have to learn how to control
your own energy.

**That's what Kundalini Yoga actually is. It teaches you to bring your transmission and your gas and your gears under your control."**

—Yogi Bhajan

The challenge is that most of us get stuck in one or two gears. We aren't able to shift the power. Think about trying to drive on a freeway in first gear only, or get up a hill in overdrive. Pretty hard, right? But that's what most of us do all the time.

When a chakra becomes unbalanced, when we block its energy from radiating and neglect its inherent talent, we can sometimes experience disease. In the three decades I have been teaching students, I've become very aware of how people inhabit their bodies, and how having emotional and spiritual "blocks" will manifest in their bodies. I can look at people and know whether they have a hard time being open-hearted to others, or whether it's difficult for them to speak up for themselves.

This book will help increase your awareness of your Eight Human Talents on a physical, mental, and spiritual level by using simple meditative and yogic techniques. And what's really amazing is that most of these little tools, meditations, and exercises take as little as three minutes a day!

The following chart provides you with a general overview of the chakra system:

FIRST CHAKRA ≋ Area of the Body: Organs of Elimination
HUMAN TALENT: Acceptance
COLOR: Red
SHADOW EMOTION(S): Resentment, Rigidity
ELEMENT: Earth

SECOND CHAKRA ≋ Area of the Body: The Sexual Organs
HUMAN TALENT: Creativity
COLOR: Orange
SHADOW EMOTION(S): Passionate manipulation, Guilt
ELEMENT: Water

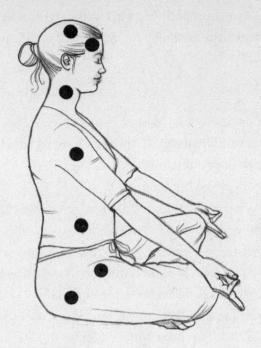

THIRD CHAKRA ≋ Area of the Body: Navel Center
HUMAN TALENT: Commitment
COLOR: Yellow
SHADOW EMOTION(S): Anger, Greed
ELEMENT: Fire

FOURTH CHAKRA ≋ Area of the Body: Heart Center
HUMAN TALENT: Compassion
COLOR: Green
SHADOW EMOTION(S): Fear, Attachment
ELEMENT: Air

FIFTH CHAKRA ≋ Area of the Body: Throat
HUMAN TALENT: Truth
COLOR: Blue
SHADOW EMOTION(S): Denial, Abruptness
ELEMENT: Ether

SIXTH CHAKRA ≋ Area of the Body: Third Eye Point
HUMAN TALENT: Intuition
COLOR: Indigo
SHADOW EMOTION(S): Confusion, Depression
ELEMENT: None

SEVENTH CHAKRA ≋ Area of the Body: Crown of the Head
HUMAN TALENT: Boundlessness
COLOR: Violet
SHADOW EMOTION(S): Grief
ELEMENT: None

EIGHTH CHAKRA ≋ Area of the Body: The Electromagnetic Field (Aura)
HUMAN TALENT: Radiance
COLOR: White
SHADOW EMOTION(S): None
ELEMENT: None

You will notice that the first five chakras are each associated with an earthly element—earth, water, fire, air, and ether. Most people recognize the first four elements, but are unfamiliar with the term "ether." Ether is a subtle, heavenly energy, beyond the earth. As we move up the ladder of chakras, into the higher mental and spiritual realms, there are no longer earthly elements associated with these chakras.

Lust, anger, greed, pride, and attachment are human qualities that result from the imbalance of the eight energy centers called chakras. When these imbalances settle in, we often experience mental or physical problems.

People often come to me with emotional blocks in a certain chakra that have manifested in the creation of a physical illness. The idea that certain emotions and talents live in certain areas of our bodies is not a new one, but I do think some people have taken this too far, and assume that if they get sick it is somehow their own fault. This is a negative way of looking at this phenomenon, and does more harm than good when it comes to healing our bodies and spirits. Your disease is not your fault. Illness is part of the whole learning experience of life, and everybody goes through it. That's what it means to be mortal.

**You can take an active, positive role in healing your own mind, body, and spirit.**

See your body as God's perfect gift to you, for it is in loving and appreciating our body that we begin the path to consciousness. The eight greatest talents of humankind are located in the eight chakras, the eight major power areas of the body. The Eight Human Talents are the gifts of God that make us different from all other creatures on earth. Happiness is your birthright. The use and cultivation of these eight talents are keys to the happiness that God wants for you.

**Happiness is your birthright.**

Our bodies are gifts from God. We need them to be here. For it is in loving and appreciating our bodies that we begin the path to consciousness. Happiness is your birthright. Opening, or balancing all your chakras is the key to that happiness.

**"The very purpose of our life is happiness, the very motion of our life is towards happiness."**
**—The Dalai Lama**

It's nearly impossible to balance these eight power centers perfectly to bring out their talents every day of your life. But don't worry, perfection isn't the goal. The goal is to become aware of the energy emanating from each chakra and to be able to call upon it when you need it. Let's say you're called on to make a presentation at a board meeting. You'll need to shift into the fifth chakra located at your throat to communicate your ideas clearly, and the third chakra to give your presentation the special emphasis and punch of commitment. If an angry coworker blows up over the smallest inconvenience, don't meet fire with fire. Try meeting her with your fourth chakra, using compassion to heal the fear and insecurity behind her outburst.

Our bodies are like complex worlds within worlds. We know where they begin and end, and yet they are vast and full of mysteries which we may never understand. No machine has ever been devised by a human that is as complex or artful as our own human body. The ancient system of chakras is a way to understand ourselves. There is an incredible amount of subtle interaction going on all the time.

I have chosen specific Kundalini Yoga exercise sequences and meditations to help you develop the human talent that lies hidden within each chakra. I suggest you choose one or two, and try them for three minutes at least. I always suggest that students begin trying any meditation for three minutes, and increase it to seven, then eleven, eventually working up to thirty-one minutes. You can see improvement by committing to doing the meditation for a longer period of time.

**"The life of a yogi is to manifest a beautiful, bountiful and wonderfully blissful tomorrow. That's a yogi."**

**—Yogi Bhajan**

The reason for these specific lengths of time has to do with the numerological significance of each number in the Kundalini Yoga tradition. The greater the amount of time, the greater the benefit. In Kundalini Yoga, we often do movements twenty-six times. Because we have twenty-six vertebrae, twenty-six is an important number to us. For a greater challenge, you can increase the number of repetitions of an exercise to fifty-four or even one hundred and eight if you really want to see faster progress!

**It's not what you do, but the courage and commitment that you bring to what you do.**

Meditation is not about perfecting or attaining anything. People think they need to go into a trance or be in an altered state to feel they're really meditating. That can and does happen, but meditation is actually the clearinghouse of the mind. Our minds release a thousand thoughts per wink of the eye. Just watch these thoughts as you might watch an ocean wave, not remembering or diagnosing them as they come and go. The real gift is to sit in the middle of all those thoughts, and react to not a one. Keep returning back to your breath, or maybe the sound you're making or the position of your body. Kundalini Meditations usually consist of breath or sound patterns and some specific positions, so you have plenty on which to concentrate.

> **"Each thought can become an emotion, and a feeling. And with each emotion and feeling, some of them become desires, and to be completed they take up all of your life energy. But if you use every thought and pass it through the intelligence and test it with your consciousness, you shall be successful, doesn't matter what. That's a simple secret of life."**
>
> **—Yogi Bhajan**

When there's an emergency—for example, if someone is calling from a hospital—we'll say, "Okay, take a deep breath, and slow down." When you don't allow yourself to breathe, you deny yourself the very gift of life. In yogic terms, we believe that the life force is the "prana," which comes to us through the breath. Allowing yourself to take in enough breath is usually the first thing you need, and it's usually the first thing to go. Breath is free for the taking, but we're often very miserly in the way we dole it out to ourselves. It's not logical, but we all do it.

Before I learned this particular technology for meditation, I experienced the frustration of being told to sit and "meditate," having no idea what that meant. I'm so glad that I now have specific tools and techniques that make meditation less mysterious and more practical.

If you want to make a real change and develop the talent in any chakra, I suggest you do a meditation for that power center for forty days, for whatever length of time feels comfortable. You can start with a shorter time and then increase the time during the forty-day period. If you just aren't up to it one day, you can go back to a three-minute period for that day so you don't have to break your forty-day commitment.

Forty days has historically been a significant time period in many world religions. In the Old Testament it rained for forty days and forty nights. In Christianity there are the forty days of Lent. Forty-day cycles are very important in the Sikh religion as well. Perhaps this is because your physical body renews all the cells in your bloodstream every forty days. For whatever reason, forty days has always been a mystical period of time.

So you see, there are many ways to use these tools. I don't want you ever to feel that the one you pick is not good enough. It doesn't matter if you do something for three minutes or for thirty-one minutes—it's all good. In this work, it is not what you do, but the focus and depth you bring to it.

Of course, it is my deepest prayer that after you do this work even on the smallest level, you will see real improvement in your life, and you will be inspired to devote more time to using these life-changing tools. In a lifetime of teaching, I have seen the technology of Kundalini Yoga and Meditation create miracles of healing. If you want healing on any level of your life and you are willing to do the work, you will see miracles, too.

## The Mystery Hidden Within Each Chakra

The first chakra, which contains the human talent of acceptance, encompasses our organs of elimination. Here we find foundation, security, and habit.

The second chakra, which contains our reproductive organs, is where we find the human talent of creativity.

In the third chakra, we come to the solar plexus area, the stomach, and many of the internal organs, such as the liver and the spleen. This area is the center for energy, for world power, for a sense of control and coordination. It is ruled by the element of fire.

Of these chakras—the first, second, and third, which make up what we call the lower triangle—the third is the most subtle. It is the driving force to act and to complete the conceptualization, the visualization that we have in our lives. It is where we find the human talent of commitment.

In the heart center, the fourth chakra, we find compassion.

The throat area, the fifth chakra, is the part of the body in which we literally "find our voice." This chakra houses the human talent of truth.

The sixth chakra is classically located at the point between the eyebrows, which yogis refer to as the "third eye point," and contains intuition. This is where we find our sense of physical vision, and our extrasensory talent of vision as well.

The seventh chakra is located at the top of the head. The exact area is where the tiny endocrine organ, known as the pineal gland, is found near the crown of the head, where the soft spot on a newborn baby's head is located. This chakra contains the human talent of boundlessness. It is the spiritual center of our physical body.

This experience of boundlessness has many names in many world religions. I chose the word "boundlessness" to describe this spiritual connection, without the specific association of any particular religion.

The last chakra encompasses what is referred to in yogic science as the electromagnetic field. It is our aura, a field of energy surrounding our physical body that makes up the eighth chakra. Western science has proved the existence of this field as a physical phenomenon. The human talent that lives in this chakra is that of radiance.

As you can see, each energy center has a profound impact on our lives. At any given time, we may lose touch with one or another of them, become imbalanced and feel "off." The purpose of this book is to find ways to connect, strengthen, and balance each of these centers on a daily basis. This process is sometimes referred to as "balancing the chakras." It is the very purpose of our lives; it is a constant and worthwhile process.

**"If you ever want to be right in your life, bring yourself into balance. The joy of life, the happiness of life, is in balance."**

**—Yogi Bhajan**

When we are imbalanced in our chakras or energy centers, we use those expressions like, "I'm having an off day," "I'm having a bad hair day," "Nothing seemed to go right today." If the chakras are balanced, you'll hear expressions like, "It was such a great day," "It was such a miraculous day. Things went so smoothly today!" And that comes when everything is lined up and the energy is flowing throughout your whole body.

Yoga is the science of breath and angles. It is an ancient science, put together by our wise elders, who were in tune with the energy field of the universe and how it manifests through our physical bodies. When we study yoga, we learn to place our arms, hands, and fingers, and the body itself into very specific postures, creating certain angles. Combined with powerful breathing techniques, these postures can produce amazing changes in our psyche!

**"Before us the sages have laid the path. We are taking our first step."**

**—Yogi Bhajan**

Yoga is similar to what keeps most animals fit. One only has to watch the stretching exercises that a cat does, and then see her magnificent body in action as she chases a bird, to understand that the systematic stretching and relaxation of our muscles can keep us fit for life.

In our uniquely human capacity to connect movement with breath and spiritual meaning, yoga is born. The translation of the word "yoga" is "union." This union of breath and movement has as its ultimate goal the harmonious merging of body, mind, and soul into the universal energy surrounding us. We refer to it as the "practice of yoga," and that is what we do in the Kundalini Yoga classes. But the *real yoga* is how you take what you've learned in class and live it out in the world.

People who are new to yoga ask me, "Is it hard? Do I have to be some kind of athlete?" Oftentimes, they give up on the very idea of yoga before they've even tried it, because they assume that it is something that dancers and acrobats do. I have students who are world-class athletes, and students who are amputees, or paraplegics, or cardiac rehab patients. Absolutely anyone can do this yoga, and everyone will be challenged by it, too. And everyone I have ever seen attempt it, even on the smallest level, has been changed. But please, if you have a medical condition, consult your doctor or chiropractor if you are unsure if your body is ready for a new challenge. Yogic technology is not necessarily a substitute for medical advice or attention; one needs to be sensitive when dealing with the complexities of the body. Once you are aware of your limitations, then be sensitive and get going!

As to "Is it hard?"—yes, it is. In various ways. Sometimes it's physically hard, sometimes it just annoys a part of your mind, what we sometimes call the "Monkey Mind." The Monkey Mind is the part of your mind that doesn't want to consider the higher questions of life. While the monkey might be asking, "Where is my next banana?" the human is asking, "Where's the next doughnut, cigarette, or mocha latte?" And the Monkey Mind will lie to you, to make sure you keep the bananas or the mocha lattes coming its way. It will tell you that this yoga you are doing is tedious, pointless, silly. Your Monkey Mind can make the yoga seem harder than it is, because it doesn't want to change.

So our Monkey Mind will tell us to turn away from things like yoga, things that portend change and seem "hard." I think we are at a point in history at which we want things to come easily. We have come to value easiness. We want a pill that will fix everything. We just want it taken care of, we want to be fixed, and we want it now. We want our lives to be pain-free, and the lives of our children to be pain-free. But what are we really looking for when we try a new diet or a new drug or a new religion? We get discouraged when things aren't easy and perfect. Kundalini Yoga can be challenging, but unlike a painkiller, it's purpose isn't to mask our pain. It *heals* our pain.

**"There is no freedom which is free."**

—Yogi Bhajan

I know, because I have been that person seeking. I spent a great deal of my life searching for the easy, pain-free fix. In my early twenties, as a flower child in the Haight, I became addicted to diet pills, because that seemed like the pain-free path to freedom. Of course, it was not.

**Pain is part of the deal.**

When I think back to that time, I was so sure someone must have the answer. I wanted someone to tell me how to make my life pain-free. Looking back, I can't imagine who I thought got through their entire lives and managed to avoid the pain. Now I realize there is not now nor has there ever been a single person on this planet who has successfully avoided the pain of being human. Pain is part of the deal.

In fact, the enlightened beings who have graced this planet dealt with the pain of humanness, and it is usually the main point of their story. This is true with Jesus, with Buddha, with Moses, with Gandhi. How did I think I could get around it?

Now since I accept pain as part of the human bargain, I am also free to accept the serenity I believe is my natural state of being. God wants each of us to live in a state of serenity. Serenity, which encompasses happiness and joy, also allows for pain and sorrow, because serenity is a state of being that accepts *all* of our states without judgment. Serenity is the state of being that exists when we are in balance, when we know our place in the universe, when we are truly able to accept God's will for us. It was the study of Kundalini Yoga and Meditation that taught me about balance and serenity, taught me how to quiet my chattering Monkey Mind, taught me how to focus on and be grateful for each breath I take.

**Kundalini Yoga and Meditation have helped me to re-pattern my body and my mind.**

As I began to learn this yoga, I began to escape the illusion I could or even wanted to avoid pain. I did begin to see pain, discomfort, and even simple annoyance, as the learning opportunities and blessings that they are. I still don't always see the traffic jam as "a growth opportunity." At first, unconsciously, I may mistake it for a complaining opportunity. And then sometimes the traffic jam, or the grocery line, or any other daily test sends me directly into impatience. I start thinking about whose fault it is that I'm stuck in traffic, or how I shouldn't have to be dealing with this. Kundalini Yoga and Meditation have helped me to re-pattern my body and my mind, so that I don't stay in the illusion of "why me" quite as long, and even when I'm in it, I remember that "this too shall pass."

This yoga can be challenging, but it can also bring such ecstasy. Once you get past the pain or the discomfort or even the simple annoyance, there can be such bliss and joy in the breath and the movement.

Someone sent me a story on the Internet that so perfectly summed up this paradox of how challenging experiences make us stronger.

One day a small opening appeared on a cocoon, and a man sat and watched for the butterfly for several hours as it struggled to force its body through that little hole. Then it seemed to stop making any progress. It appeared as if it had gotten as far as it could and it could go no further.

So the man decided to help the butterfly. He took a pair of scissors and snipped off the remaining bit of the cocoon. The butterfly then emerged easily. But it had a swollen body and small, shriveled wings. The man continued to watch the butterfly because he expected that, at any moment, the wings would enlarge and expand to be able to support the body, which would contract in time. Neither happened!

In fact, the butterfly spent the rest of its life crawling around with a swollen body and shriveled wings. It never was able to fly.

What the man, in his kindness and haste, did not understand was that the restricting cocoon and the struggle required for the butterfly to get through the tiny opening was God's way of forcing fluid from the body of the butterfly into its wings so that it would be ready for flight once it achieved its freedom from the cocoon.

Sometimes struggles are exactly what we need in our life. If God allowed us to go through our life without any obstacles, it would cripple us. We would not be as strong as we could have been. We could never fly.

I asked for Strength . . .

And God gave me Challenges to make me strong.

I asked for Wisdom . . .

And God gave me Problems to solve.

I asked for Prosperity . . .

And God gave me Brain and Brawn to work.

I asked for Courage . . .

And God gave me Danger to overcome.

I asked for Love . . .

And God gave me Troubled people to help.

I asked for Favors . . .

And God gave me Opportunities.

I received nothing I wanted

I received everything I needed.

I just love that story, because I asked God for a way to avoid pain, and God gave me Kundalini Yoga.

As you begin to read, know that each of these eight energy centers already lives within you, each of the chakras is like that butterfly trying to be born out of its cocoon. The whole process of learning is really the process of uncovering and rediscovering what we already know. That is the process we will undergo together.

I know by the end of this journey we will see our eight glorious human talents begin to thrive. We humans are magnificent creatures. This is the perfect time for us to celebrate and nurture our Eight Human Talents together.

Our bodies are the means by which we come to know and understand our spiritual connection to the Infinite. John O'Donohue, gifted poet of the spirit, sums up this relationship beautifully in the Celtic poem from his book *Anam Cara: A Book of Celtic Wisdom*.

## A BLESSING FOR THE SENSES

May your body be blessed.

May you realize that your body is a faithful and

beautiful friend of your soul.

And may you be peaceful and joyful and recognize

that your senses are sacred thresholds.

May you realize that holiness is mindful, gazing,

feeling, hearing, and touching.

May your senses gather you and bring you home.

May your senses always enable you to celebrate the universe

and the mystery and possibilities in your presence here.

May the Eros of the Earth bless you.

# 1
# The First Chakra

**"The first chakra represents the earth element, the strength, the grit, that bullish part of you."**

—**Yogi Bhajan**

The first chakra is the realm of habits, the land of automatic behavior and deep instinctual patterns we learn for survival. It is at the very base of the spine, the power center that comprises our bowels and our anus. Just as our arms and hands are associated with the heart chakra from which they emanate, so are our legs and feet related to the first chakra. It is our unconscious center, deeply shared across all of us, regardless of intelligence, status, or age. The character of the first chakra is to "reduce everything to the bottom line."

**"First you make habits, then habits make you."**

—**Yogi Bhajan**

The color that is traditionally associated with the first chakra is the color red. It is the flash point of the eternal flame burning in our first three chakras, which combine to make up what is called the "lower triangle." It can be the red of the burning ember at the center of a roaring fire, or it can be the musty red of clay, or the deep crimson of a ruby forged by pressure deep within the earth.

We connect to the planet through our first chakra, and it's where we return ourselves back to the earth beneath us. It is at our first chakra that we accept we are even here on earth. It is where we first say "yes" to life.

**"If the roots aren't deep, the tree can't stand the weather."**
**—Yogi Bhajan**

A student told me a story recently about a conversation she had with her brother. They have always had a strained relationship, which she attributes to the fact that they grew up in a home with an alcoholic father. This girl's brother never wanted to admit that fact, and often ridiculed her for trying to heal herself about this issue.

She wanted to accept her father. Her brother didn't even want to admit there had ever been a problem, and he resented that she constantly kept bringing up the topic. She wanted them to talk about their father and his drinking, but eventually stopped trying. She felt her brother never talked about anything real. As a result, their relationship was always cordial, but not close. She longed for this closeness, especially after the death of both her parents.

Recently her brother was going through a difficult time with his own family. When other people suggested that events from his past might be affecting his present, he began to listen. As often happens, being in the middle of an emotional crisis opened him to a deeper level.

He began reading literature about adult children of alcoholics, and identified with what he was hearing. What his sister had talked about all those years suddenly started to make sense. It had been decades since he had spoken to his sister about these issues. He decided to call her to talk about their father's drinking.

She was surprised and happy to receive his call, and hear him say he was beginning to understand their father had been an abusive alcoholic. The conversation was important for both of them; they both expressed acceptance for each other and for their father. The brother was beginning to understand what their father had done to them, as well as why, and that brought understanding and acceptance to him. For the first time in decades, this student feels as if she may be able to feel close to her brother. Such is the awesome power of acceptance.

**Acceptance opens us up physically. The tightness in the lower back frees up, the clenching in the lower intestines loosens.**

I think this is why the story of the prodigal son has always been one of the most popular biblical stories. Another version of the theme of the prodigal son is a story that appears in a wonderful collection of inspiring true stories. In this story, a young Jewish son decided to rebel against his father. He did this by renouncing their Jewish faith, which the father treasured dearly. The son resented the fact that his father would not let him choose his own spiritual path. In turn, the father resented his son's refusal to honor their religious tradition. His father had been a Holocaust survivor. He had pledged that the religion for which his relatives had died would be honored in his family. When the son turned his back on their faith, the father turned his back on the son, disowning him and banishing him from the family home.

Having wandered and traveled for many years, the son ran into an old friend who told him that his father had just died of a heart attack. The son was overcome with grief and guilt, because he was certain that he was responsible for his father's broken heart.

The son was tortured by one thought: if only he could turn back time and tell his father that he loved him, and beg for his understanding. But of course, that was impossible. Feeling lost and alone, the son decided to go to Israel, to the Wailing Wall, where Jews have for centuries gone to petition for miracles. The son wanted to go there to pray for his father's understanding, even though it was too late.

When the son arrived at the Wall, he recited the long-remembered prayers his father had taught him. Then he prayed a prayer of his own, begging for his father to understand that he had loved him, and that he was sorry for the pain he had caused him. He looked around and saw that other petitioners were writing notes and placing them in crevices in the wall. He was told that people wrote down their petitions and placed them in the Wall, praying that this place was so holy that prayers were granted in miraculous ways.

The son, like the others around him, wrote a note. He asked for his father's understanding, and told him that he loved him, that he had always loved him, even when his father had banished him from the family home. The son took the note and tried to find a place to put it in the very crowded wall. When he finally found a spot, and squeezed his missive between the tiny cracks in the stones, another note fell out. When he opened the note that had fallen into his hands, a miracle did in fact occur. The note was in his father's handwriting, and it was written to his son, telling him he loved him, that he had always loved him, even when his son had turned his back on their faith. The acceptance of each other's paths and lives, which both longed for, had been granted.

The miracle in the story is not that the two men placed notes in the same tiny hole in an ancient wall. The miracle is that these two men were able to overcome their own wall of resentments, and allow themselves to share in the healing miracle of acceptance.

In order to truly accept, we must make our peace with our own human nature. It is here, in our first power center, that we must accept our own existence. If we are balanced in this part of our body, we feel at home in our own skin, we feel cozy and secure and that it's okay for us to exist on the most basic level. If we don't feel supported, grounded, comfortable in our own skin, we are likely to be filled with resentment.

**If we don't feel supported, grounded, comfortable in our own skin, we are likely to be too full of the shadow emotion of this chakra, resentment.**

People steeped in bitterness and resentment are miserable, and yet a part of them remains firmly attached to their own misery, because at least it is familiar. Who is to say that getting rid of misery won't just make room for a newer, bigger kind of misery? It's the old dilemma of the devil you know being somehow better than the devil you don't know.

We have recently opened Golden Bridge, our new yoga center. We found a five-thousand-square-foot building, gutted it, and began designing and rebuilding—a dream come true. I was working in a group, managing every single detail of the Center. Since a director had not yet been appointed, a lot of time was wasted in circular discussions in which no real conclusions were reached, which was challenging for all of us.

Eventually the group decided that I would be the director of Golden Bridge. I was frightened and not sure if I was up to the demands of the position. As God will do, the Creator gave me an opportunity to heal this insecurity: My lower back went out. I was flat on my back and in a lot of pain; even getting up to go to the bathroom was agony.

It happened in the middle of teaching a pregnancy yoga class. I didn't want to alarm the women who were resting and meditating at the time. So severely had I displaced my back that I couldn't move, and wondered how I would even get to a seated position so I could finish out the class and send my dear moms-to-be on their way.

I had ten minutes to do it. I took a full agonizing ten minutes to crawl back to my pillow. After class was over, my husband carried me out of the Center and drove me home, where I lay in bed for about a week. Lower back pain, I learned, is one of the main reasons that people are absent from their jobs.

It was physically and mentally painful, but I knew this was a moment of demarcation—a big change was on its way. Though I was scared and in so much pain, a part of me was excited and trembling. I prayed and prayed and prayed—not to release the pain, but to understand what I needed to learn from this event.

There were three other times in my life that this happened to me. The first time, in my early thirties, I was supposed to be the maid of honor at my roommate's wedding. I felt I was losing my best friend and that scared me. I felt abandoned.

My back went out, and I missed the wedding. Her husband-to-be was a chiropractor. An hour before the wedding, he came to our apartment and tried to treat me, with no luck. Finally he had me on the living room floor, packed in ice. I could not move! At the time, I had no clue about the connection between mind and body. Twenty years later, they still kid me about it.

The second time was after the birth of my daughter. All of my fears about the health and well-being of my daughter came up. At one point in my life, I had had a son who died seven months after childbirth. After I lost my son, it had taken me twenty years to get pregnant, and I was scared she would have the same destiny.

Number three was when my mother was dying. She was ninety-two years old, and her death was a very healing experience for all of her children. She was simply fading away from old age, preparing to leave gracefully, and we were helping her. At my sister's home in Gainesville, Florida, I would get into bed with my mother, cradling her in my arms as I know she cradled me as a baby. She wasn't always aware of what was happening, but there were beautiful moments of clarity. I held her small, frail, slender body and we talked about how she was going Home, and she said she wasn't afraid. I told her it was okay to go, and she repeated back to me that yes, it was okay to go and that she wasn't frightened of death. I would lie with her and she would recite after me the Twenty-third Psalm, line by line, "The Lord is my Shepherd. I shall not want." I stayed with her several days and then went alone to India, where my daughter goes to a boarding school. I was going to teach the children; I knew I would not see my mother on this earth again. I left her in the care of my sister, Ana Marie, who is a healer and one of the kindest human beings on the planet. I knew Mom was in God's hands.

I took off for India. Crossing Europe, I had a strange feeling in my lower back. I hadn't experienced this much pain in more than thirteen years, since my daughter was born. My eyes were burning and itching as

I had never known. I continued my journey feeling it all would pass, but instead it only increased. By the time I landed in Delhi, I could barely walk or see. I was scared. How to carry everything to the train station? I had so many extra duffels of children's Christmas presents. I put on a pair of sunglasses and took the journey inch by inch, step by step. Porters helped me, and I got on the train, going north for six hours. It took fourteen hours because of a railroad strike in Ludhiana. Due to a labor dispute, the train stood still for six hours in the middle of nowhere. There was fighting at the station. Many jumped off the train and made it by other means. I could go nowhere, because by this time I could barely walk or see. I could go nowhere, so I sat, meditated, and prayed. My mind went off to my mother. I knew she was almost leaving.

Finally the train moved, the fighting ceased, and we could pass through the station. We arrived at two A.M. at the ancient train station in Amritsar. My dear daughter and her friends were awaiting me in a horse-drawn rickshaw. During the next four days, I lay still at a guest house with my eyes closed. I could not move or see. Yet, somehow I wasn't worried or scared. I knew my mother was dying, and there was a part of me going out with her. The pain was my body's way of honoring the gift she had given me—life.

On the fourth day, my daughter came after school and said, "Mataji" (which means Beloved Mother), "Auntie called and said Grandma left her body." I lay there very still, uttering the sounds of "Wahe Guru" (which translates, "Great is the ecstasy of God's Creation"). My daughter lit a candle and we chanted together five times, "Akal." It means "undying," and is what we sing at the time of someone's death, so they may be returned Home. We offered it to my mother so she might leave easily, fearlessly, and gracefully. Within two days my back and eyes were returned to their usual health and strength. I never tried to figure it out, just as I don't try to figure out many things in life. It's Guru's grace, God's grace—"Ek Ong Kar Sat Nam Siri Wahe Guru," as is said in the Sikh scriptures. "There is One Creator who has created this creation. Truth is The Creator's Name. Great is The Creator's Wisdom."

My sister later told me my mother left her body very peacefully. She simply took her last breath and then breathed no more. My sister was right there in bed with her, and continued to hold her for a very long time, feeling the warmth slowly leaving our mother's body. I am grateful for so many things about my mother's death. I am grateful that she was peaceful. I am grateful that she was surrounded by love, and that we had so much time to talk and say good-bye.

The remembrance of things past had stirred up old pains and unresolved conflicts. Just the idea that my mom, the one who had given me life and sustenance, would no longer be there for me, brought up to the surface fears of survival. This all resulted in a weakening of my lower back once again.

**It's only when you truly surrender and accept that can you move on in your life.**

In each of my incidents of back pain, I can remember the exact moment that it started to go away, and that was always when I began to surrender and accept myself, my family, and my life. Then I could move on. By the fourth time this happened, I knew right away I needed to accept myself, and everyone else.

**"It is in Pardoning that we are Pardoned."**
**—Saint Francis of Assisi**

I am grateful for all the backaches. Each of them gave me the gift of trust and acceptance. When I look at any time I have had "dis-ease" in my body, I am grateful because they have been learning opportunities— although it's sometimes difficult to see in the pain of the moment. In the three back experiences, I was learning trust. Trust in God—God is the Doer of everything. If you find yourself in the situation of experiencing an extreme amount of back pain, the most important thing you can do is nothing. This is particularly hard for most of us. We like to fix it *now*. The old aphorism, "Don't just do something—sit there," really applies in this case. Eventually the spasm will lessen. If you push it, if you don't listen to your body, you will only compound the problem.

## CORPSE POSE

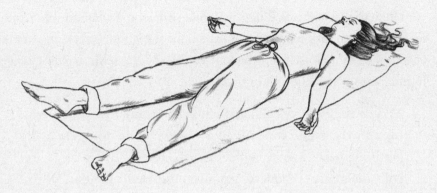

What you can do is meditate. There is a pose in yoga that is referred to as "corpse pose." It consists of lying flat on your back with your legs stretched flat, and your arms by the sides of your body, palms open and face-up.

This is a posture we assume at the end of every yoga class. You can cover your eyes with something to block out the light if you want. Wrap yourself in a warm blanket, and if you're feeling weak in your lower back, place a pillow under your knees. When you are lying in corpse pose, you can inhale and exhale very slowly through your nose. This is a great opportunity to observe and connect with your breath, because even without trying you will automatically be breathing from your belly.

## ROOT LOCK

Another technique you can add is the practice of pulling the root lock, or *mul bandh*. Contract the muscles of the anus, sex organs, and navel at the same time. (Note: If you are in the first three days of your moon cycle don't do this lock. Also, if you are pregnant, isolate and squeeze only the first and second chakras.)

The best way to do this is to complete a full cycle of inhaling and exhaling through your nose. When you are completely emptied of all breath, it is then you pull the root lock and hold it for a few seconds. After that, let go of the root lock and begin to inhale once again. Keep your eyes closed and rolled upwards. See how long you can hold the root lock before you take in another breath. This small internal exercise helps you to pull up energy from the earth itself. *Mul bandh* builds a strong foundation in your body and mind.

> **"When the energy of the first chakra is stimulated and distributed to the body, you will find a newness in you. Then the earth element, the strength, the grit, the bullish part of you will come alive. Whenever you need the earth element, all you have to do is mentally squeeze this area. Then you can be on top of yourself. Your own chakra will serve you."**
>
> **—Yogi Bhajan**

The most enduring image in Kundalini Yoga is that of the snake. The word "Kundalini" is defined as prima energy that rests at the base of the spine like a coiled sleeping snake. We begin to awaken this coiled serpent of energy, and as the coil unwinds, it begins to spread its energy up and down the spine. To do this is referred to as "raising the Kundalini." It's a beautiful image when you consider how mysterious the working of the spine is. As those who have suffered from spinal cord injury can attest, the spine and how it functions remain mostly unknown to modern science.

EXERCISE
SPINAL FLEX
Finding where we hold deep insecurities that might be decades old, even as far back as life in the womb, and beginning to release them on a

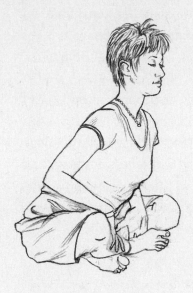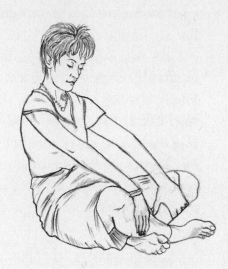

physical level can be a catalyst for incredible emotional transformation. If there is an old insecurity that makes you tense up just thinking about it, find a way to clear it, or it'll eventually make you sick.

Try this exercise as a starter:

1. Sit in easy pose with your legs crossed, resting comfortably on the floor.
2. Hold the ankles with both hands, and deeply inhale.
3. Flex the spine forward and lift the chest up.
4. As you exhale, flex the spine backwards.
5. Keep the head level so it does not flip-flop.
6. Repeat one hundred and eight times, or for about three minutes.

*Effects*: Spinal flex in this position stimulates the first chakra, releasing tension and channeling energy up the spine, as well as balancing the lower organs. You may notice that you feel calmer and more centered after doing this exercise.

**"Just meditate on the first chakra, just feel it. If one can feel it, one can stimulate the seventy-two thousand nerves located here**

in no time. The moment you concentrate on it, the spinal fluid starts flowing directly through the gray matter of your brain."

—Yogi Bhajan

People often say to me that they would like to be more accepting, but they just don't know where to start. Yogi Bhajan, my beloved teacher, says, "Fake it and you will make it." Acceptance is one of those things. Take the action—the feeling and the healing will follow. If we wait for the perfect moment to accept someone, it will never come. If we wait until we are no longer bothered by someone's behavior, there will never be any acceptance. Acceptance is an act of pure grace.

**Acceptance is an act of pure grace.**

Doing yoga and meditation prepares us to open up and accept on a daily basis. Doing something as small as inhaling deeply, holding the breath, and then pulling the root lock makes us feel more grounded. When we are grounded, we aren't afraid and insecure, and are more capable of accepting.

**When I am grounded, I am more capable of doing the big emotional work of acceptance. Acceptance is the opposite of judgment.**

## Breath Work to Build Trust

Another simple reminder is to spend one to three minutes concentrating on exhalation. Inhale deeply through the nose, and then exhale through the nose every last molecule of air. Experience what it means to give everything away.

**Trust at its most elemental level is an act of giving.**

Only when we are willing to give away every last particle of breath, which is our life force, can we truly receive. My teacher, Yogi Bhajan, reminds us that when you give as much as you can of yourself, the universe then rushes in to fill the vacuum you have created. The body provides a tangible example of that: When you empty your lungs, you must trust that in the next instant, you will inhale and be filled with air. All the inspiring words in the world cannot teach us as much about giving as truly exhaling all the air in our lungs.

A few weeks ago I attended the Los Angeles Festival of World Music. The opening event was at the Hollywood Bowl, and His Holiness the Dalai Lama spoke. There were musicians from every part of the globe. The music was inspiring and transcendent. As always, His Holiness's presence was inspirational. His words of compassion and acceptance filled thousands of people's hearts with a sense of hope for real world peace. I remember leaving the theater and feeling myself in a warm cocoon of bliss from the music and the wonderful words he had spoken. It had been a long concert, and we were happy but tired. I had the sense that every single one of the thousands of people who were streaming out of the amphitheater had somehow been altered by the whole event. There was a powerful feeling of serenity in the air. A feeling of total self-acceptance, self-respect, and self-love seemed to permeate the crowd, as evidenced by the smiles and kind gestures all around.

**Becoming aware of your body through yoga and meditation is the first step to accepting your body.**

The expressions people use when they talk about non-acceptance tell us a lot. We talk about "carrying a grudge," "being trapped in the past," and "being full of bitterness." All of these images evoke a sense of physical bondage or suffering. As long as we live in non-acceptance, we are under the power of fantasy. Often without being aware of it, we let a false image of another person control our lives because of our inability to accept that person. It is a cycle that only we can stop.

"To carry a grudge is like being stung to death by one bee."
—Anonymous

Acceptance is a major tenet of almost every major world religion. Jesus said, "Father, forgive them for they know not what they do." Jesus was a master of acceptance and understanding. This was one of the pivotal messages of his teachings that two thousand years later we still hold as true.

On a theoretical level, acceptance is a great and noble ideal. Though many people might agree that acceptance provides great benefit to us, they may not understand that there's a physical price to be paid when we choose again and again to live in resentment and judgment. Living in judgment will manifest in our bodies in the form of illnesses.

**If you accept and learn not to criticize yourself, you will find true health—physically, mentally, and spiritually.**

Digestion and elimination are often the source of concerns that keep many people from feeling fully healthy on a daily basis. You need only to watch a few hours of advertising on television to see there are a lot of people in this country having problems in these areas.

Many studies have proven that regular physical exercise is an important component to healthy digestion and elimination. Our Western diet of refined foods with little or no fiber content is also a culprit. Digestion and elimination troubles can be solved without artificial laxatives or other digestive medications. With yoga and meditation, a positive mental attitude, and lots of fresh fruits and vegetables, healings take place. If what you eat does not eliminate within eighteen hours, it poisons your body.

EXERCISE
SQUATS, OR CROW POSE
One very basic yogic exercise that can work wonders is a simple squat. The West has lost the art of squatting. Just as white bread became what the

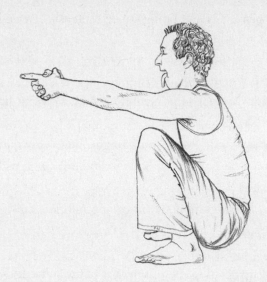

European upper classes ate while brown bread was left to peasants, squatting became what peasants did while higher classes sat in chairs. That is how the spine began to deteriorate. Everyone, even the very oldest people, used to squat to cook, sweep, eat, chat, and even eliminate. Today, though squatting to go to the bathroom is not practical for most people, given the setup of most modern plumbing, doing squats on a daily basis would do more to help people's digestion, elimination, and spine than any of the hundreds of digestive remedies and tonics you can buy at the pharmacy. We do a squat in Kundalini Yoga in what is known as "crow pose."

1.    Place your feet shoulder distance apart or a little wider. Ideally your feet would be pointing straight ahead, but if it helps to have them angled out, that's fine. For many people who are not instantly able to do this move, placing your back against a wall and sliding down into the position can be helpful.

If you are feeling shaky, you can also place two chairs, one on either side of you, for support. It doesn't matter what it takes to get you into the squat. Just get yourself there and you will reap great rewards.

If you can only go halfway and be on the balls of your feet, start there. Inch by inch, you will become a squatter and you will feel so much better.

2. Once you get into the squat, extend your arms out in front of you, with your hands clasped together.

3. Stretch your index fingers out straight, as if you were pointing towards some distant spot in the horizon.

4. Keep your eyes one-tenth open and pick a spot in front of you to stare at in order to keep your balance.

5. Open your mouth, extend your tongue, and begin panting through the open mouth as you pump your belly in and out along with the breath. This is similar to how a dog pants.

6. Begin by holding the position for one minute, and work your way up to three minutes.

*Effects*: This posture opens up the entire base of the spine and connects you to the earth. It strengthens your legs and thighs as well as your rectal muscles. Eventually you'll find this pose to be quite relaxing. Oftentimes in India, we see people sitting in a squat for sheer comfort's sake.

Squatting is a very natural way for human beings to sit. It is the ultimate ergonomically designed chair.

Once you are in this pose, this would be a great time to meditate on those people in your life you want to understand and accept, trusting in life and God, and leaving all judgement behind.

Acceptance of someone does not excuse their transgressions. It just means that you don't want to be burdened with the feeling of the pain it caused any longer. You accept another to set yourself free from the bondage of resentment.

Here is a beautiful story of acceptance. A group of Tibetan monks were making a sand mandala as part of an exhibit on Tibetan culture. A sand mandala is a very intricate religious painting laid out on a floor, made up completely of colored sand. Part of the beauty of the art form is that it is, by its very nature, impermanent. After the mandala is consecrated in a ceremony, it is dismantled. Finally, the wonderfully colored sand is collected together and then deposited into a body of water.

This delicate mandala was being laid down in San Francisco. The monks had been meditatively and diligently working on it for days. Suddenly with no warning, a mentally disturbed person came running through the room and destroyed the mandala, kicking the sand with her feet. In a few seconds what had taken days to create was gone.

Patrons of the museum and other passersby were very disturbed by the event. Many were even moved to tears. On the other hand, the monks, from the depths of their total "beingness," simply accepted the situation, and began to rebuild the mandala. Acceptance and respect of all sentient beings is a central component of Buddhism. They saw that the woman was in a great deal of pain to commit this random act of violence, and needed their understanding. They simply smiled as if the mandala had not been disturbed, and began the work of rebuilding.

As long as we deny that we have anything in common with the person we are resenting, it will be impossible to accept him or her. If, instead, we try to imagine what the other person is feeling, we find that the iron chains of resentment automatically begin to loosen.

Empathy is not sympathy. Sympathy says, "I feel as you do," whereas empathy says, "I know how you feel." The best part of empathy is that it allows for healthy detachment. I don't need to feel your suffering, I just need to remember that I, too, have suffered as you are suffering. Empathy is about acknowledging that we are all separate, but also interconnected.

One student, a waitress, has told me how impossible some of her customers can be. She described one customer, a very well dressed businesswoman who would come to her restaurant for lunch almost every day. She usually dined alone, reading business reports and annoying others by chatting loudly on a cell phone. Everyone in the restaurant called her "Mrs. Cranky," because the woman was always returning food, complaining that a draft was blowing on her, and often seemed to take it personally if the restaurant had run out of a particular item. She thought nothing of berating the waitress for things that were clearly not her fault. My student dreaded waiting on her, but the woman kept coming back.

One day, Mrs. Cranky came to the restaurant, accompanied by an ancient woman in a wheelchair who was obviously her mother. On that particular day, the persnickety customer was very quiet. All her usual complaining behavior was being taken over by her even more persnickety mother. The mother was more impossible than the daughter had ever been, and berated the entire wait staff. Her own daughter seemed to become like a shy, insecure five-year-old, completely powerless to stand up for herself. She hunched over in her chair, almost as though she were cowering from someone who was about to hit her.

The student saw all this, and began to have empathy for Mrs. Cranky. Seeing how she had been treated all her life made it obvious why she felt the need to treat others so abusively. She decided that she would commit to ending the cycle of abuse. From that day forward, she treated this annoying customer of hers with love, kindness, and understanding.

The ending of the story is not what you would expect. The customer did not soften under the constant barrage of kindness that emanated from the student. Instead, she seemed distrustful and annoyed. It was almost as if she felt that the kindness she was receiving was a trick. Mrs. Cranky was putting out hostility and by God, she expected hostility to come right back. That is how she had been raised. As unpleasant a life as it was, it was clearly the only way of being she could understand.

Eventually, Mrs. Cranky stopped coming to the restaurant altogether. The student says that although the customer didn't respond to her kindness, she herself got an enormous benefit from altering her behavior. She said, "I just felt lighter. I have always dreaded waiting on that customer, and suddenly I found myself looking forward to it. It made me feel so good about myself that it didn't really matter what the response was. I didn't care if she liked me. I liked me." That was the real gift that came from putting compassion into action.

The waitress saw another human being as the frightened and confused child she once was. When you find yourself reacting to someone's behavior, the first thing you can do is to imagine that person as a seven-year-old. The man waving his fists at you in traffic is really nothing more than a little boy whose father doesn't have time for him. The rude clerk at the DMV is really nothing more than an ashamed little girl who's been told over and over again that she is ugly and stupid. If you take the time to see the hurt and sorrow, it becomes easier to have compassion and move on with the rest of your day.

**To live without compassion is to take on a physical burden. Poison seeps into every cell of our body and very often the disease that results is cancer.**

Top cancer researchers have tried for years to figure out what makes a normal cell suddenly become cancerous. The answer is yet to be found. The idea that non-acceptance is the trigger that causes healthy cells to mutate is as plausible as any other explanation.

**"Without Forgiveness, Life is Governed by an Endless Cycle of Resentment and Retaliation."**
— Robert Assagioli

A high school teacher described a wonderful exercise she used to teach her students about acceptance. She had gotten the idea from another teacher and has used it with her students every year since. She tells the students to bring a clear plastic bag and a sack of potatoes to school. For every person they judged and could not accept, they would take a potato, write that person's name on it, and put it in the plastic bag. She told them to be sure not to leave anyone out. Everyone who had ever done them wrong needed to be in the bag. By the end of the class, most of the kids had bags that were full to overflowing. They were then instructed to carry the bag with them everywhere for one week, putting it beside their bed at night, or on the seat next to them on the bus. They were never to let the bag out of their sight. If another member of the class saw them without their bag, they would get an automatic "F" for the assignment.

By the end of the week, the students were sick to death of their bag of resentments. It was annoying having to lug them everywhere. And on top of that, the potatoes themselves had begun to turn moldy and stinky. The students' bags of resentments were heavy and awkward and seemed to be making their lives miserable. The teacher then told the students that carrying the potatoes was a wonderful way to understand the price we pay for hanging on to resentments.

Fortunately, when the week was over, they were free to put down their sacks of potatoes. She suggested to them that the lightness they now felt, the feeling of freedom at not lugging that heavy sack, was only a taste of what they would feel if they would actually accept and let go of judgment and resentment for each person a potato represented. The burden of carrying their resentful feelings was so much heavier than the weight of one small potato ever could be.

> **"Love yourself. Love your soul and let go of the past. Past pain is keeping you in pain. You don't have to deteriorate."**
>
> **—Yogi Bhajan**

A student shared with me a story about the transformational effect that the attitude of acceptance has had on the life of her family. She has two daughters. Although both girls are out of high school, they continue to live with her. She is a widow, and grateful to have her two girls at home.

Her oldest daughter is a constant thorn in her side. They have always had a difficult relationship, and they nag at each other constantly. The mother would feel terrible for the way she would criticize her oldest girl, and yet five minutes later the girl would do something to annoy her, and they would be at it all over again. It usually would start over something small, like leaving dirty dishes in the sink, or forgetting to walk the dog.

She began to ask herself, "Why am I so hard on this child? Is it because she reminds me so much of myself at her age?" She was thinking about this on the day before her daughter's birthday, and came to the realization that she preferred the company of her youngest daughter. She didn't know why she preferred her, she just did.

It was easier for her to love the baby. If she just admitted the truth of that, maybe she could find a new way to love her eldest. She wondered, did she pick on her oldest girl because she was not as easy to love as her easygoing younger child? She realized it wasn't so much that she needed to accept her daughter for all the annoying things she did. She really needed to accept herself for not loving the elder girl as easily as she loved her baby.

She decided that on her daughter's birthday, without telling the girl, she would vow not to criticize her even once, the whole day. No matter what happened, she wouldn't say a single negative thing to her daughter. It would be her way of accepting their relationship.

For the entire day, she managed to not say one critical thing, although she certainly found this very difficult. When her daughter wore ripped jeans to the nice restaurant they went to that night, she wanted to say something and yet she didn't. When the girl didn't react in exactly the right way to a certain gift she was given, the mother wanted to scold her, but she left it alone. That night she went to bed feeling very proud about the secret gift she had given her daughter, one that her daughter didn't even know about. It had been one of the nicest days she could remember their spending together in a very long time.

The next morning she woke up and thought, "You know, that went so well, I could actually extend the secret gift for another day, just to see how it goes."

She knew that eventually she would have to criticize her, say something negative, but it would be kind of a challenge to see how long she could keep it up. She certainly couldn't expect to keep it up forever, but it wouldn't be that hard to do it for just one more day. When that day had ended, she decided to extend the gift to the next day, and then the next.

As of today, she has kept it up for six months. The transformation in this relationship has been miraculous. Before, they often spent days in sullen silence, but now they seem to enjoy each other's company. As an additional side benefit, the dirty dishes and the un-walked dog seem to not be a problem anymore. More often than not, her daughter takes care of the things she is supposed to do automatically, no nagging necessary. What's even more of a miracle to this student is the fact that on those days when the dishes are left behind, it just doesn't seem to bother her anymore. It's as though her obsession with her daughter's faults and shortcomings have been lifted from her. When she tries to work off her old patterning, it simply isn't there.

**True acceptance can transform our lives.**

By accepting herself, and asking for the acceptance of her daughter, not with words but with actions, this student has transformed one of the most important relationships in her life for the better. This story reminds me that actions speak louder than words.

**Acceptance is one ingredient in the recipe for transforming your life.**

Just as the first chakra is at the base of our physical body, so is acceptance at the base of our spiritual body. It is where it all begins. Researchers who have done personality inventories on groups have determined that people who are more accepting have better physical health, and more long-lasting relationships. They have found no such positive benefits for non-acceptance. They have found no such benefits for holding grudges.

> "There is God—
> Where all men of all faiths,
> All flowers of all colors and different fragrances
> Care to get together.
> Let your bouquet live; Let your soul prosper."
> —Yogi Bhajan

If you begin your day in acceptance and thankfulness, you will follow in the path of some of the greatest people who have ever lived. Buddha, Mohammed, Jesus, Guru Ram Das, the Dalai Lama, Yogi Bhajan, Martin Luther King, Mother Teresa, every admirable person you can think of was gifted beyond compare with acceptance of all.

> **"If you can't see God in All,**
> **Then you can't see God at all."**
>
> **—Yogi Bhajan**

If you can accept another, you will be able to accept yourself, and you will find a lightness in your life that is beyond compare. Resentments will be lifted, and you will become aware that we are all interconnected. You will begin to feel acceptance resonate within you, within your cellular structure.

## "Let Go, Let God"—A Mantra of Acceptance

As you go throughout your day, become conscious of your breath. Let your exhale be a physical letting go, and as you become aware of that letting go, silently chant on every exhale, "Let go, let God." You don't need to analyze this process—just trust it. Go through your day, silently repeating the phrase, "Let go, let God."

Accept your parents, your siblings. Accept your spouse, your relatives, your teachers, your boss. Accept your children, understand and accept the first person who broke your heart. Accept the last person who insulted you. Understand and accept yourself—for *everything,* including not being able to accept some people just yet. When you are ready to, you will, and when you do, you will receive a feeling of lightness of being that you never dreamed possible. You will be in a state of grace.

Allow yourself the precious rewards you will be given if you choose the human talent of understanding and acceptance on a daily basis. Do it for this one day only. Tomorrow you can decide if it is worth doing again. And remember, it all begins with self-acceptance.

"There is nothing good, nothing bad—thinking makes it so.
Think deep. Think good.
When you think big, you become big."

—Yogi Bhajan

Your body is your temple, and the quality of your choices create the structure of your body, mind, and spirit.

FIRST CHAKRA EXERCISES
MOVING CROW POSE

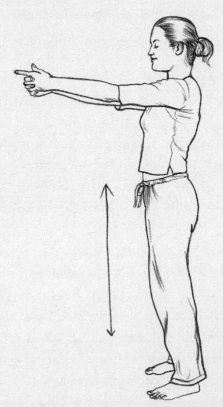

1. Come into a squat, as explained earlier in this chapter.
2. Place your hands straight in front of you, parallel to the ground,

elbows straight. Clasp your hands with the index fingers pointing straight ahead. Keep your elbows straight the entire time.

3.   Inhale through the nose, and push off the earth using the force of your heels, coming up into a standing position, straightening the knees. The arms are still parallel to the ground.

4.   Exhale through the nose, and come back down into a squat or as far as you can come down.

5.   Inhale as you go up, mentally reciting "Sat"; and exhale as you go down, mentally reciting "Nam."

6.   Keep your eyes one-tenth open.

7.   Repeat anywhere from seven to twenty-six times.

*Exceptions to this pose*: Women who are pregnant or on the first three days of their period should not do this posture.

*Effects*: This posture is very strengthening, both physically and mentally. It stimulates the energy of the first chakra and then brings it up your spine. It can help strengthen your leg muscles, and improve your posture. Plus it grounds you to that place of total self-acceptance.

BODY DROPS

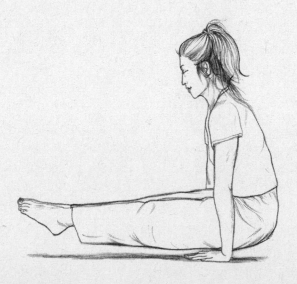

1.   Sit on the floor with your legs out in front of you.

2.   Place your palms flat on the floor, fingers pointing forward, on either side of your buttocks. If your wrists are weak, do it with your hands in fists.

3.   For just a few seconds, lift your entire body off the floor, and then drop yourself back onto the floor. If you can't lift the entire body at once, go for the buttocks first, and then lift the legs—like a rocking horse effect.

4.   Work it up to three minutes.

*Effects:* If you do this for even one minute, you'll usually feel the beginning of an emotional release. People worry they might injure themselves, but in fact this movement is very safe. Once you get over the reaction of the sheer silliness of it, you might find this is an exercise you'll begin to crave. I like to do it with some kind of very high-energy music playing, coordinating the rhythm of the movement to the beat of the song.

## MEDITATION FOR REJUVENATION

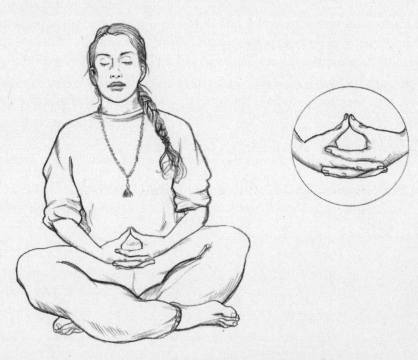

1.   Sit comfortably in a cross-legged position on the floor (easy pose). If this is not possible, you can sit in a chair, as long as both feet are flat on the floor and the knees or ankles are not crossed. Sit with a straight spine, and pull the chin slightly into the chest.

2.   Close your eyes and bring them to focus at your third eye point, the point between the eyebrows, in the center of the forehead.

3.   Interlace your fingers and press your thumb tips together firmly. Place your hands in this position in your lap with the palms face-up.

4.   Apply *mul bandh* by contracting and pulling up on the rectum and sex organs, and pulling in on the navel point, all at the same time.

5.   Keep this contraction and pull on all three centers as you inhale and begin to chant aloud, "God and me, me and God, are one."

6.   Exhale. Release the contractions. Then inhale deeply a second time, and repeat the sequence from number five above. With each repetition of this mantra, pull up on the locks a little tighter.

7.   Continue for three to eleven minutes.

*Effects:* This meditation can improve your health by invigorating the first chakra and elimination organs. It promotes calmness and disease resistance.

Squeezing the anus, if done properly, can invoke the earth element, and can bring about a renewed sense of strength, grit, and determination. Whenever you are dead tired, or feel you are about to fall apart, apply this lock. It will help you to go solidly through everything.

**"If a person can apply root lock, he becomes invincible."**
—**Yogi Bhajan**

# 2
# The Second Chakra

CREATIVITY

"Whenever you do something, do it as a piece of art. Otherwise just don't do it. Let everything express the creativity of you."

—Yogi Bhajan

Each chakra is a vision of the world. It is a collection of our feelings, thoughts, and values, and how we encounter the world within them. The second chakra is about desire, passion, duality, polarities, movement, change, and creativity. In the body, it is related to the area of the reproductive organs. The second chakra invokes so many contradictions in us. Our entire economy seems to be fueled by this center, and yet people do not associate the idea of sexuality with creativity. Those who function strongly out of this center move at a speed dictated by their feelings, desires, impulses, and passions.

Unlike the first chakra, for which the vision of the world is singular and isolated, the energy of the second chakra involves other humans. When your second chakra is well developed, you have opinions, make distinctions with passion and motivation. Your language, when motivated from this center, is sensual, glorified, flexible, directed with a goal. It is the center that opens you for merger, dissolving your sense of identity into another human.

Life, when you are vibrating positively from this center, is colorful, vibrant, and deeply meaningful.

When a person is blocked in this center, life is listless, empty, and the world is tedious and boring. When this chakra is overstimulated, the person sees everything in terms of sexuality. Everything is said or done with one goal in mind: to try to fulfill the person's passionate nature.

Marketing experts have concluded that in the course of a day the average American sees thousands of advertising-related images, and a great many of these are sexual in nature.

Advertisers are not interested in appealing to our creative sense of sexuality; mostly they are interested in making us feel inadequate, with the idea that purchasing their product will somehow remedy what is wrong with us. Cars, phones, beverages, shoes, whatever they are selling, if you buy it, you will be sexually desirable.

The reason that all of this has such a powerful pull on us is that marketers are hitting on a basic truth: As human beings, we are by our very nature conscious of our sexuality. We alone among the animal kingdom worry about our sexuality. We are also the only animals that have the knowledge to make decisions about our own reproduction. Members of the animal kingdom certainly exercise choice, but we are the only ones who consciously delay or reject the notion of having offspring.

The power we have over our own procreation is an awesome power, but like all leaps in consciousness, there are costs to this power.

For example, if lions thought consciously about their sexuality, they could be made to feel insecure about it. Other lions could convince them that they would only get a mate if they had a full beautiful mane, and the jungle would be echoing with the sound of lion-sized blow dryers. As it is, we are the only creatures that give our sexuality that much thought.

**Human beings are the only consciously sexual creatures and as a result we may be the most sexually insecure creatures on earth.**

In the classical system of chakras, this second power center represents more than the creation of human life through reproduction. The second chakra is said to govern all areas of human creativity. We are also alone in the animal kingdom as the only creatures who become aware at an early age that we are mortal. The decision about what to do with our finite time on earth is the biggest exercise in creativity that can be made, and we get to revise that decision every day, every moment of our lives.

The color associated with this chakra is orange, the color of tigers, and pumpkins, and copper, and tropical fish. It's a bold color no matter what the hue, a color that demands attention. You can't ignore orange.

The element is water. Water doesn't have a set shape and neither do emotions. Someone who views the world primarily from the second chakra sees everything as a sexual object. In reality, it's much bigger than this. *All* liveliness and movement of life comes from the energy of this chakra.

Generally, people associate "creativity" with artists; in actuality, creativity is everyone's birthright. It is the act of living here and now, finding out what it is that makes you happy, and then pursuing that path or way. It involves discovering what it is that you genuinely love to do, and allowing it to manifest in your life.

Your creativity, like every one of your human talents, is a direct gift from God.

**"Creation is only the projection into form of that which already exists."**

—**Shrimad Bhagavatam**

I like what Julia Cameron has to say about creativity in her classic book, *The Artist's Way*. She wrote, "Creativity is like your blood. Just as blood is a fact of your physical body and nothing you invented, creativity is a fact of your spiritual body and nothing you must invent."

**"To live a creative life we must lose our fear of being wrong."**
**—Joseph Chilton Pearce**

Living a creative life may include artistic endeavors of the traditional kind, but it is time for us to expand our notions of what is creative and valuable. One of my students, whose mother is a well-known artist, has great respect for her mom's work as an artist and teacher. She remembers the small ways her mother brought creativity into their lives—her endless display of art on the walls as though their house were a gallery. She remembers her mom's ability to create a beautiful centerpiece out of a bowl of pebbles.

Of all the artistic works her mother created, she remembers most the inventive way her mom would cut their sandwiches in three parts so they resembled angels, with a cookie for the head. When she describes these "angel sandwiches," her eyes light up with the delight of a five-year-old. The sandwiches her mother made or the pumpkins she carved were never reviewed in the *New York Times*, but they all add up to a creative life, lived by a woman who had an abundance of creativity. She did what she liked and she found her happiness there.

**To experience true creativity, we must always be willing to let go of the results, whether it's a novel or our children.**

We often think in order for a creative effort to be worthwhile, it must have some chance at permanence. But to experience true creativity, we need to let go of the results, whether it's our novel or our children. Ultimately, what we have a hand in creating exists on its own. It's easy to see that is true with an herb garden, but it's much harder with a child. As a parent, I understand the desire to try to control our children's choices.

**A good way to begin developing our second chakra of creativity is to begin physically.**

**"When the body is in rhythm, there is ease. But when any part of the body goes out of rhythm, there is dis-ease. Disease is nothing but an out-of-rhythm body."**

**—Yogi Bhajan**

I see many students holding a tremendous amount of tension in this chakra. Resentment and blocks in this area can lead to serious consequences, as do all psychic blocks. Among the "dis-eases" that manifest in the second chakra are menstrual difficulties, infertility, kidney and bladder problems, prostate cancer, ovarian cancer, hormone imbalances, and many more.

EXERCISE
PELVIC TILTS
A wonderful beginning exercise for opening up this chakra is one I love to do first thing in the morning.

1. Stand with your feet shoulder distance apart, feet straight forward, and legs slightly bent. Rest your hands on your thighs, right above your knees.

2. Press your chin into your chest, allowing your whole spine to curl up, with your pelvis tipping forward.

3. Then reverse the movement and lift your chin out and up, allowing your pelvis to tilt back. In other words, stick your behind out, tipped up.

4. Inhale through the nose as the spine goes forward, and the head and buttocks are up. Exhale through the nose as the chin tucks in, and the

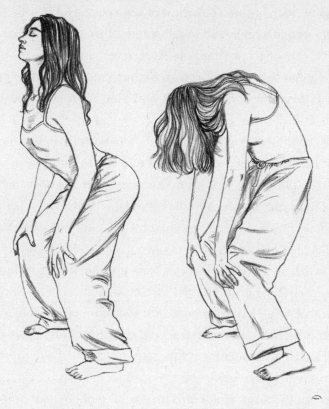

spine arches high. Allow the breath to be long and deep. Do this for one to three minutes.

*Effects:* The movement is small and easy. Do it and you will see how it generates heat in your second chakra. This is an exercise you can certainly do for as little as one minute and feel a real difference. It's a great one to do if you are in the middle of such creative things as composing a symphony or reorganizing your sock drawer. You will find that just one to three minutes of this will reenergize your effort.

This is also a great exercise to do if you are having a difficult menstrual period. In Kundalini Yoga, we alter the way that we exercise during menstruation. This is not meant as any kind of judgment on women—in fact, quite the opposite. This form of yoga honors the fact that the bodies of women have a special and exalted task, the ability to conceive and bear children. During this time, many exercises are modified. We don't do anything that puts excess strain on the second chakra.

The power of childbearing is one that has special meaning for me both as a mother and as a teacher.

My daughter, Wahe Guru Kaur, was born in 1984. I was forty-two, and at the time that was considered quite late in life to bear a child. I had also had a child as a very young woman. My baby boy was born with a congenital heart defect. After living in the nightmare maze of the medical system at that time, he ultimately died after only seven months. My experience of childbirth had not been a happy or empowering one. I was never allowed to make choices about my method of birthing, medications, or anything else. That, of course, was the rule and not the exception at that time. Even my desire for something as simple as not having him circumcised was overruled by the authoritarian male doctors who thought they were in charge of us both.

This experience was profound for me. It galvanized me as an advocate for mothers and children. The teaching of pregnancy and post-natal yoga has become a major part of my life's work. I like to think I honor both my daughter and my little son with the work I do with pregnant mothers.

I tortured myself—as do most parents who have children that are born with medical problems—wondering if it was my fault. I was left with years of guilt and self-doubt.

Guilt is one limited emotion sometimes associated with the second chakra. For me guilt is summed up in the idea that I am "less than."

Yogi Bhajan says, "Faith is something someone else tells you, and guilt is something you tell yourself."

Creativity is the talent that most resonates with all our issues around money. Survey after survey indicates that the two most common problem areas in relationships are money and sex. Welcome to the second chakra, home of money and sex, where there is more than enough guilt for everyone.

## FLOW

Money is a symbol for the nectar of life. If you are the rare person who was raised to love yourself and honor others, you probably don't have issues around money.

Having a healthy attitude toward money issues is related to the idea of flow, and that is one reason that money is also referred to as currency. Money needs to flow, like a current, in order to function optimally for all of us. It's an elegant spiritual principal and a practical economic reality.

The second chakra is associated with the element of water.

A practical way to remind yourself about the importance of allowing money to flow naturally in your life is to remember to drink a lot of water.

If you find yourself in a place of terror or guilt about money, make sure that you are drinking enough water. It's practical health advice you've heard thousands of times, but how often have you resisted it? The number one reason I always hear is, "Because I hate having to go to the bathroom all the time."

Begin to acknowledge the flow within your life. We are beings who are more liquid than we are anything else. We need to hydrate and urinate. Consider the idea that if you aren't hydrating your body, chances are that you will be in a dry spell financially as well.

I have received many lessons about money lately. Here is an example: I had been teaching yoga in my home for a couple of decades. I never really advertised, I never had to pay rent for a business space, employ other workers, apply for licenses—none of that. I just taught in my living room, and people put their money in a jar on my hall table, and it worked out very well. I also taught private sessions to people in their homes. I went on like this for many, many years, perfectly content, and God always provided.

Then in my meditation, God spoke strongly to me. *More people need to experience Kundalini Yoga and Meditation. Now is the time.* If a person is really sick mentally or physically, I still see him privately, and give him a *sadhana* (a personal self-practice) and then find other healers or practitioners to help him along. I help people individually who are committed to practicing on their own, but I realized that my teaching would be mostly with groups. I believe in what Jung calls the "collective unconscious."

**When we gather to do yoga in a group, there is a healing wisdom that benefits everyone who participates.**

I know that leading people in this way is my true calling. So I made what seemed like a difficult economic decision: I would give up my private teachings, and teach group classes only. Some of my private clients were not pleased, but many of them understood my decision, and have continued their practice on their own and by coming to class. I thought that perhaps I would not make enough money, but I left it to God. Almost immediately, my classes started getting larger. In fact, they got so large that they began to be too big for my little house. I prayed for guidance.

**God often sends us angels in the disguise of troublemakers.**

God sent an angel my way in the disguise of a nosy neighbor who decided to call the city's zoning department. To my surprise, I discovered, after decades of teaching, that it's actually illegal to teach yoga in your home in Los Angeles. I thought it was a crazy law, but realized that fighting the city wouldn't solve my problem, because I had too many students for my house to hold anyway.

**"In creating, the only hard thing is to begin."**
**—James Russell Lowell**

So my husband and I decided to open a yoga center. What had been a very simple proposition—you come, I teach—evolved into a giant undertaking with architects, workers, insurance, permits, bylaws, finding a location, and all the rest of it. As anyone who has a business can tell you, it is quite overwhelming—and that I was. I wondered if we could handle it. How would we get enough money to complete the work we needed to do? Would people find us? I prayed more than ever and kept turning it over to God. My husband and I went through so much in our relationship. Trust in God and the creative force of the universe kept us going.

**If we see ourselves as living in a universe of plenty, we will be more willing to share, and then there will be plenty for everyone.**

When I had taught in my own home, we had always served yogi tea (cardamom, ginger, peppercorns, cloves, and cinnamon all boiled together to create a wonderful brew) and cookies after class. Kundalini Yoga is so powerful, and brings about such expansive mind changes, that when you finish class you need to ground yourself. To connect back to the earth and earthly things, we relax after class with a cup of yogi tea and something sweet.

There was a lot of discussion about the "tea and cookie issue." A number of people felt that it was too complicated to do in a larger center. It would be too much work, it would be too expensive, we couldn't afford it. Someone even suggested that we charge for the tea and cookies, which I was adamantly against. My initial feeling was, if we could afford it when there were fewer students, why couldn't we afford it when there were more? But I was not confident of my opinion, and let the issue slide in the rush to open the new center.

I felt the idea of not enough money to pay for tea and cookies was coming from a place of contraction rather than expansion. If we see ourselves as living in a universe of plenty, we will be more willing to share, and then there truly will be plenty for everyone. If we see ourselves as living in a universe of poverty and lack, then we will tend to hoard, and there will not be enough even for ourselves.

Every student who came to the new center asked about the tea and cookies—"Will there still be tea and cookies?" The custom represented real nurturing and coziness to the students. I had to speak up on this issue, and find a way to keep the yogi tea and cookies as they had always been—free and plentiful. We found a way to bring giant pots of yogi tea to the center on a daily basis. We began to order cases of health food cookies, wholesale. We found a graceful way to serve all this after every class, and it has worked out just fine. Now, watching students sipping tea and nibbling on their cookies as they share each other's company makes my heart so happy. And not surprisingly, business at the center has been growing steadily.

**Our personal financial abundance should be a direct result of our viewing everything as a gift from God.**

There is a real imbalance in our society about sex and money. Our personal financial abundance is a gift from God. Everything is created by the Creator. Our finances, our work, our families, all of it.

This seems logical, and we want to believe it, and then you look at the fact that some of the wealthiest people we can think of are not spiritual or generous at all. They have created wealth, but have never left their second chakra and connected with their hearts. So how can having personal abundance be related to our acknowledging the presence of the divine in everything we create? That is a good question, and there's a real simple answer. You must define your terms. If you define abundance in numbers, then what I say will not be proven true. If you define abundance in terms of feeling there is plenty, then this view of it is right.

**If you define abundance in terms of feeling there is plenty, you will be rich every day of your life.**

The chakra system helps us to understand our bodies. Metaphors are important; they bring understanding. When we marry we say that, "The two shall be as one." Obviously we don't mean they are now conjoined twins connected by living tissue. We mean it as a metaphor. That's why the metaphor of partnership, two halves of a whole, can help create a healthy marriage, or heal an unhealthy one. For that same reason, we can view our body as comprising eight power centers. Imagining each center exuding one of the brilliant gifts or talents of humanity can help us create a metaphorical self-image of our physical body that is physically healthy, happy, and whole.

The Divine Mother, the nurturer of the child, the earth itself, is becoming more present in the West. We need the Divine Mother energy to balance out the predominant male energy. Both energies are needed for balance. Both need to be honored.

This shift is happening at Golden Bridge, our new center. We are starting to get more and more male students. There was a time when classes would be overwhelmingly female, not due to any effort or plan on our part. That's just the way it was.

There have been periods of time historically in which women were prevented from practicing yoga. Happily, that idea is mostly a thing of the past. In the last few years, I have seen a dramatic increase in the number of men in my classes—often there is an even fifty-fifty split. Men are courageous enough to accept a woman as their teacher, they are willing to bypass the huff and puff of the gym for a mind/body/spirit workout.

I also see revolutionary changes between men and women in the pregnancy and post-natal classes I teach. Fathers are more actively involved in the birthing of their children.

It's hard to imagine that as recently as twenty years ago having a father in the delivery room was quite uncommon. Now it is rare *not* to have a father present at the birth of his child. That is a quantum leap in consciousness, and I can't wait to see what this generation of babies who are welcomed to the planet by both their parents turns out like. They will surely help lead this earth to peace.

**A generation of babies who are welcomed to the planet by their parents will lead this earth to peace.**

I am very optimistic about our evolution of sexual consciousness, but I have to acknowledge that we still live in a time of incredible sexual wounding. Though abuse that was once hidden away is being exposed, and given a chance for healing, we are far from living in a society where people are safe from sexual predators.

Many people are also confused about what comprises healthy sexuality for themselves. Outdated rules have been swept away, but there isn't a code of sexual ethics to replace them yet. We have sexual freedom, but we're not entirely sure what to do with it.

When I was young, I created mental imbalances with excessive sexuality. I look back and see that much of my longing had to do with the loss I felt after the death of my baby and my father. I attempted to erase the guilt and grief I felt by acting out through promiscuous sex. I had indiscriminate sexual encounters. It took work to develop a sense of balance about my sexuality. The good news is that I am now a post-menopausal woman who takes no hormones, and I have never felt more beautiful or sensual in my life.

I know from my own difficult experience that doing Kundalini Yoga and Meditation led to my sexual healing.

I respect every woman's choice to accept or reject hormone replacement therapy, but I do see the one-sided sell job many doctors give to their patients. Certainly a long-living population of women on synthetic hormones represents a large profit for the medical establishment. There may be women who would do best on this therapy, but medicine seems to regard menopause as a disease instead of a natural path to wisdom.

When I went through menopause I did my yoga and meditation as always, I used wild yam as a supplement to ease any discomfort, and I continued to eat soy products and yams (which have natural estrogenic compounds) along with my vegetarian diet. I used no hormones, and my health and enthusiasm for life have remained alive and well, the best ever in my life.

I am not desperate to pretend I am a thirty-year-old woman. I am not, and I couldn't be happier about it. I am fifty-seven, and I feel very blessed.

Maybe it's because I live in Los Angeles and am surrounded by so many people who work in the entertainment industry, but a large number of students worry about their age. A student who is an actress came to me almost in tears because she was suffering terrible menstrual cramps. I talked with her a little bit about this, wondering if there might be some sort of emotional component to what she was feeling on a physical level.

She told me she recently turned twenty-five, and was sure her chances to pursue her art were now over. She didn't come up with this idea on her own, she had been told by her agent she "only had a few years left." I found this notion insane, and told her so.

She was "trying to be realistic about her chances," and I believe that her agent's words—and more important, her acceptance of them—were an assault. Although I am not in her business, I know that great success in any business is based on people believing in themselves and in their creativity. In all lines of work, there are certain accepted "truisms" that are proven to be false every day.

**"Be realistic—plan for a miracle."**
**—Bhagwan Shree Rajneesh**

Another woman I know wanted to be a doctor, but she was discouraged because she was in her thirties. Another wanted to get her Ph.D., but thought it was "too late." The whole issue of age hits women particularly hard because of the time limits that exist in our bodies for fertility. Do not be limited by age, even in the area of raising children. I had a child when I was forty-two, and have seen other women defy the odds in the fertility arena, or choose to adopt.

A student I love dearly is forty-five and pregnant with her first child. She came to my Kundalini Yoga classes after trying many fertility treatments. She was desperate to have a child. We talked about this, and she agreed to commit to a regular practice of yoga and meditation and prayer.

She did her yoga and meditation for three years, with no result—no result in terms of pregnancy, that is. Her overall health improved, she reached an optimum weight with which she was comfortable for the first time in her life, she stopped having panic attacks, and on the rare occasion that she still had them, she knew how to calm herself by using the curled tongue breath meditation. She came to peace with the idea that she, at age forty-five, was probably not going to have a child of her own. She and her husband began to talk about adopting.

**"I do not believe in miracles, I rely on them."**

**—Yogi Bhajan**

I'm sure you can guess what happened next. She became pregnant. She was deliriously happy, and has been a picture of health throughout her pregnancy. She tells me she is sure she became pregnant precisely because she stopped trying to get pregnant. Doing a practice of yoga and meditation allowed her to relax and trust in a way that had never been possible for her.

Anyone who works for a baby doctor or an adoption agency can tell countless stories of couples who couldn't have children until they relaxed and surrendered. Oftentimes the pressure to produce a baby is off when a couple adopts, and often the mother becomes pregnant after years of trying.

This notion has been borne out in recent research on infertility. A study done at Harvard Medical School showed that women who went through a ten-week stress-reduction program conceived at a forty-four percent higher rate than women who didn't.

Of course, there are times when this kind of story doesn't end in a pregnancy. I have worked with many couples who became parents through adoption. I have seen many happy endings, or I should say beginnings. To those who feel there should be some set limits on the age that people can conceive or adopt children, I do not agree. If the parents are committed to a healthy lifestyle, people have the capacity to live long enough to become parents at almost any age. I have seen people who do yoga and meditation in their eighties run circles around unhealthy people in their thirties.

## SEXUAL ADDICTION

Another kind of sexual healing seen among our yoga students involves those who have been sexually addicted. A gay man in his forties came to me a number of years ago. He was involved in a long-term relationship, but there were difficulties, particularly in the areas of money and sexual fidelity.

This student and his partner both started doing yoga. Although they were both incredibly fit, they found the yoga challenging, more so on a mental and spiritual level. They were unused to connecting with their spiritual side through movement. They did not come to a yoga practice expecting to have it help them with their relationship problems, but that is ultimately what began to happen.

The original student ended up not staying with his partner, but continued coming to yoga alone. I gave him a forty-day meditation to practice. He began to do some serious self-examination, particularly in the area of the second chakra. As a result of his deeper commitment to his yoga practice, he came to the conclusion he had a sexually addictive personality, and it had been a large part of the problem in his relationship. He decided to seek help for this pattern of behavior with therapy and by participating in a twelve-step program.

A gifted designer, this student was abundant with creativity. He also seemed to have a disproportionate amount of the corresponding shadow emotion of guilt. Although he thought he was very open about his sexuality, he realized he carried a lot of guilt, not necessarily sexual guilt, but guilt in other areas of his life.

He had his own business, and often worked long, arduous hours, not taking time to rest or eat properly. He often found himself as a caretaker, and more often than not, picked lovers who were financially dependent on him. All of this came from an overwhelming sense of guilt that he could not really define. He began to face up to the fact there was a part of him that liked playing the role of the martyr. If he was doing "too much" for someone else, it would put him "above criticism."

He had grown up in a household with a father who was verbally abusive and relentlessly critical. It wasn't too hard to figure out from where that relentlessly critical inner voice was emanating. This newfound realization didn't turn him against his father. Ironically, it planted the seeds of understanding, allowing them to mend their relationship before his father died.

As he continued his yoga practice, his therapy, and his twelve-step work, he found himself making more aware choices. These good things he was doing for himself sustained him through a very difficult time. Within the course of a few months he simultaneously lost his father to cancer and a dear friend to AIDS.

During that difficult time he began a small yoga class for people from his support group, teaching them the yoga and meditation that had helped him so much. He found this was a way of giving and nurturing others that was appropriate, not martyr-like, and as a result he got as much from the teaching as his students.

## BALANCING AND HEALING OUR SEXUAL INJURIES

The desire to reclaim our self-worth is a common response to sexual abuse.

It often manifests with very controlling behavior around sexuality, either through promiscuity or frigidity, both being manifestations of the need to have some sense of sexual control.

Students find serenity and balance in their sexual lives as a result of doing yoga and meditation. Doing this work allows the body, mind, and spirit to balance and harmonize itself.

Our culture's images of sexuality have created a wounding in many people—the idea that a man's status and worth are derived by the number of women he can bed, and the corresponding idea that a woman is valued by the affluence and power of her partners. Popular culture is a reflection of our own values. A nighttime soap about the lives of a contemplative religious order entitled *Monk's Place* would not get the same ratings as *Melrose Place*.

If the media you choose to watch and consume don't reflect your core sexual values, they ultimately are not healthy for you. Be mindful about what you choose to watch and read. Surround yourself with images that are nurturing and sexually healthy. One way I accomplished this in my own life was by taking a little corner in my new house and making it into an altar. Our house was built in 1922 and has not been changed at all. There is a hallway niche which in the twenties would have housed a phone and a little chair. I built an altar with all those things I love to look at—pictures, photos, flowers, silks from India, candles, incense, and lots of color. Rose petals from the Golden Temple, holy water from Italy, two stones from Tibet, and shells from Greece also adorn this sacred space.

I keep a candle lit for a particular prayer I may be having—for the healing of someone sick or my daughter who has just gone back to India, a pet that's disappeared, or someone's mother who has just died. It is one of the last things I see before I blow out of the house on a busy day, and it reminds me of what I hold as the highest ideals.

## KUNDALINI YOGA: THE YOGA OF AWARENESS

Creatively choosing what images we are surrounded by increases awareness.

The Tibetans are very visual when expressing Buddha nature, or God. Their temples and religious costumes are all balanced with color and symmetry for the eye to behold. They meditate on hand-painted mandalas. By staring at one in meditation, you can come to know God. We have many mandalas in our house and at the yoga center.

**Connect your creativity to God, to your higher self, and you will begin fully to experience this human talent of creativity.**

Love to live creatively. Become conscious of the creative choices you can make on a daily basis, and infuse them with meaning.

Become aware of your surroundings. Maybe it means spending more time in the produce section of the grocery store, really noticing the dizzying variety of fruits and vegetables that are gathered there, the pretty way they are stacked, the juxtaposition of the colors and shapes.

Children do this easily. All of this might seem childish, and that is exactly the point. "Only as a child shall you enter the Kingdom of Heaven." Recovering your creativity often means taking a little trip back to the time of life when it was abundant in you. It's important to connect with that place inside us that loves to watch the play of colors on a soap bubble, or wants to learn to whistle through a blade of grass, or listen to crickets.

Kundalini Yoga is often referred to as the "Yoga of Awareness." Creating a shrine or altar is a part of my yoga practice.

When teaching a class, I ask my students to smile. The physical stretch of the smile becomes part of the posture. Yoga is an awareness applied to action.

Another tool to find your optimal sexual health is a forty-day celibacy. This would mean not having sexual contact with others or with yourself. Celibacy can be a form of meditation, although it's not terribly popular among students. Students who have consciously committed to this discipline, and have shared their thoughts with me about it, said they thought it was very valuable for them.

One benefit of a forty-day celibacy is that it makes you more aware of how you use your sexual energy in your life. Do you use it for sacredness, or just as an outlet to release excess energy? A person may find during the forty days that he's addicted to sexuality, that it's an addictive behavior. You never really know until you take something out of your life, take a vacation from something, exactly how it fits into your life. Once the "vacation" is over, you reenter with a fresher, more aware state of mind. For people who have made sexual activity a routine, one that has lost its zip, they can reenter the experience more meaningfully. When you are in a relationship, it's a good thing for both of you to abstain, because you find other ways to express your love and other ways to become close. And other ways to work things out, as well. Instead of fighting and making love as a way to make up, discovering more healing ways to come back together is very valuable.

If you take up this practice for a forty-day period, it will be most valuable if you keep a journal of your feelings. A great time to do this is at the end of the day. Just commit to writing one page longhand about what you are feeling. You don't have to go back and read it—just the act of writing down your thoughts and experiences will be enough.

When it comes to your sexuality, the awareness and action are up to you. Leave guilt behind. Turn instead to self-examination, and then action to change that which is unproductive for you and your fellow humans. Seek out help and counseling if needed.

Guilt has its purpose. Just as anger, fear, and grief have their appropriate places, so does guilt. Allow guilt to serve as a warning for you; let it tell you when you are violating your own core values. If I am on the phone with a maddening bureaucrat at the phone company, and I speak harshly to that person, as I did recently, I feel guilty. I get to take a look at that, and wonder if that fits into my highest ideal for myself, and then I get to call that person back and apologize. But that is where the guilt ends. I don't have to keep track of my bad behavior and use it to beat myself up. I took care of it, end of story.

If we don't use guilt as a warning device the same way we use fear or anger, it begins to fester in us, and robs us of our creativity.

As a teacher, I am truly blessed. When my spiritual teacher, Yogi Bhajan, came to America in 1969, he came not to gather students, but to create teachers. He has done that on a worldwide level, developing teacher training programs throughout the world. We at Golden Bridge have our own nine-month training program for anyone who wants to learn in-depth and teach.

One of the most honored ideals of Kundalini Yoga is service. When you find techniques in this book helpful, pass them along to another.

Many people who learn even one posture, breathing technique, or meditation might think to themselves, "I am not a yoga teacher." However, if you teach even one little exercise to another in need, that is exactly what you are.

If you teach a frightened child how to take a deep calming breath, or if you show a tired clerk how to refresh his mind by closing his eyes and rolling them upward, you will have given them the gift of self-healing. As a result, you will begin to understand that gift more completely for yourself. As they say in many twelve-step programs, if you want to keep the gift, you have to give it away.

**"If you want to know a thing, read that. If you want to understand a thing, study that. And if you want to master a thing, teach that."**

**—Yogi Bhajan**

There is an exercise that is so simple and feels so good. It is exactly the kind of exercise anyone could teach to almost anyone. It has the added brilliance of being the sort of thing you can do while sitting at your desk, really almost anywhere you have the chance to sit quietly for even thirty seconds. It is nothing more than a simple pelvic rotation.

EXERCISE
PELVIC ROTATION

1.  Sit on the floor, preferably with your legs comfortably crossed. If that's not possible, you can be seated in a chair. Close your eyes and turn them toward your third eye point.

2.  Place your hands around your kneecaps, and start moving your entire upper body in a circle, making a grinding motion in the pelvis, as though you were some kind of human mortar and pestle. Your legs and your buttocks would be the mortar, and the rest of your body is the pestle, slowly rotating your upper body in a clockwise direction.

3.  Continue churning in the same direction for one to three minutes, and then reverse the motion and churn in the other direction for approximately the same amount of time. As you go back, the chin tucks slightly into the collarbone. As you go forward, the chin extends with a stretch through the throat. Since Kundalini Yoga is all about balance and union within ourselves, be sure to repeat it going in the other direction the same amount of

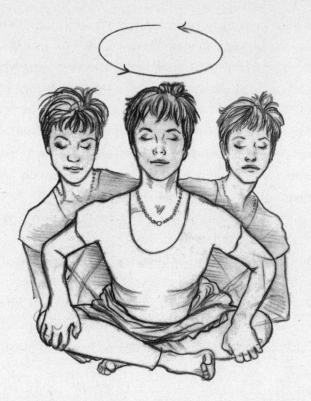

time to get the full benefit. Even if you do the movement for only a few seconds, be sure to repeat it going the other direction, so you get the full benefit.

4.   The breath is long and deep, inhaling as you rotate forward, exhaling through the nose as you rotate back. This breath pattern has an almost instantaneous calming effect on most people, which is why this exercise is very powerful, despite its apparent simplicity.

If you choose to deepen the benefits you get from Kundalini Yoga by sharing it with another, this is an ideal exercise with which to start. I have never met anyone who couldn't do it. We often use this as a first warm-up exercise at the beginning of class, before the actual *kriya*, or set of exercises.

Sharing with others is part of what the energy of the second chakra is all about. Creativity involves us with other humans. Creation of life through our sexuality involves interaction with another. Being human means we must necessarily depend on another to create new life.

Beyond this simple fact, most creativity involves interaction with our fellow humans. Although we can create for our own enjoyment, our work and our artistic endeavors are richest when we share them with others. If no one is an island, it is mostly due to our need to create.

Naturally these sorts of time-wasting opportunities are liable to be presented to you with alarming regularity if you are fortunate enough to be a parent or to have spent time with children. It is often a challenge for high-achieving adults to find an interest in collecting rocks with a four-year-old. Perhaps by shifting your perspective, and giving yourself over to this seemingly mindless pursuit, you will discover it is exactly what you need to kick-start your adult-level creativity.

Sometimes I have yoga students take a walk during class. They pair up and one student closes her eyes, while the other leads her by the hand outdoors. With eyes closed, they touch everything, feeling the textures of leaves, walls, bark, whatever there is to be touched out there in the big wide world. Creativity begins with the sense of touch.

### HAUNTING THOUGHT MEDITATION

One way that's easy to end the guilt cycle is to do a meditation at night, in which you exhale away those things you feel guilty about from the day. It takes only several minutes.

This meditation can cure phobias, fears, and neuroses. It can remove unsettling thoughts from the past that surface into the present. And it can take difficult situations in the present and release them into the hands of Infinity.

1. Lower the eyelids until the eyes are only open one tenth of the way.
2. Concentrate on the tip of the nose. Silently say, "Wahe Guru" in the following manner: "Wah"—mentally focus on the right eye. "Hey"—mentally focus on the left eye. "Guru"—mentally focus on the tip of the nose.
3. Remember the encounter or incident that happened to you.
4. Mentally say "Wahe Guru" as in number two.
5. Visualize and personify the actual feeling of the encounter.

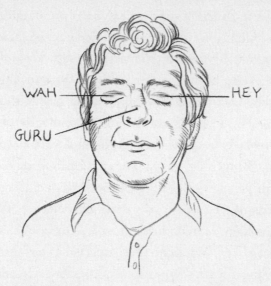

6. Again repeat "Wahe Guru" as in number two.
7. Reverse the roles in the encounter you are remembering.
8. Become the other person and experience that perspective.
9. Again repeat "Wahe Guru" as in number two.
10. Forgive the other person and forgive yourself.
11. Repeat "Wahe Guru" as in number two.
12. Let go of the incident and release it into the universe.

These are twelve steps to peace, given by Yogi Bhajan. Share them with a friend!

Intense guilt or regretfulness is an extreme form of self-hatred. It is the voice that says we will never be attractive enough, smart enough, good enough. When this self-hatred becomes more than we can bear, it gets turned outward. Every act of rape or sexual violation is self-hatred turned outward on another. Most of us have felt self-hatred at some time in our lives. Although most people don't act it out in these horrifying ways, we identify with the core feeling. That is why crimes of sexual victimization bring out so much revulsion in us, because on some level we identify with the core feeling, if not the action itself.

I had a student who admitted that he was a pedophile. He wanted to learn how not to act out on his compulsions. At first it was difficult for me to relate to him. I respected him for having the commitment and courage to seek help, and I felt called to help him as best I could. I put it to prayer.

I asked if he would be willing to meditate every day and attend class three times a week. He agreed, and faithfully began showing up. He was involved in intense counseling, and the yoga and meditation helped him to understand where he had gotten stuck. He did a lot of second and fourth chakra work. As the power centers are linked, the work benefited his whole being. By opening his heart center, he took the focus from his obsession with the shadow side of his second power center.

Guilt was one of the primary triggers in his behavior. When his self-loathing became overwhelming because of his unacceptable desires, he was tempted just to say, "What the hell!" and to act on his compulsions. Instead of using his guilt as a warning alarm, it became an eardrum-splitting siren to run away from as quickly as possible. Once he ran away from his guilt on a metaphorical level, he felt free to victimize others. Guilt so out of balance did not inhibit his actions.

He began to explore other, healthier, areas of creativity, including his yoga practice. Instead of losing himself in forbidden desires, he lost himself in the elegance and challenge of a posture, the constant vastness, capability, and endurance of his body, and the deepening of his ability to find release in meditation. As a result, he felt calmer and stronger, both physically and mentally. He was beginning to accept a divine presence in his life, and found himself relying on the presence of God to remove his compulsive behavior. Today he is no longer a sexual predator.

This student reminds me that "God and me, me and God, are One." By opening ourselves physically, mentally, and spiritually to that power that is both within us and beyond us, everything and anything is possible.

**We are born out of a moment of creativity.**

Against great odds, one sperm out of millions penetrated one egg, at the exact moment of ripeness. It is a miracle. You are a divine Creation. Every human being has a divine purpose, something that you and only you are here on earth to give. It might be a monument, or a discovery, or a simple act of kindness that unknowingly transforms the life of someone else.

In 1976, I had a great sadness so overwhelming I felt that I could not live through it. My ex-husband had left me, and our spiritual group, in New Mexico. He just walked out, never to return. I wandered the cornfields every night. In order to stay alive, I would go into a fantasy and say to myself that when I went to sleep, I would awaken in the morning and everything would be just as it was before he left. And that's how I survived without dying.

One day a friend found me wandering in the fields. What she said that day has stayed with me forever and helped me through that valley of darkness. She said, "You know if you left, you would be missed, for there is no one on the earth to take your place. We all have a part of this whole, each one of us." These two little sentences stuck with me and got me through this period of my life, and still does. My spiritual teacher sent me to India to visit the Golden Temple, where a healing took place.

Chances are there are many things that you will be called to create in this lifetime, and it is never too late to begin. You can begin to create your life with your next breath, or the next one after that. The choice is up to you.

If you keep up, you will be kept up. If you give up, God can do nothing. So, KEEP UP!

## Second Chakra Exercises
## Frog Pose

1. Come into a squat, up on the toes, pressing your heels together. Have the knees bent and spread apart, and the buttocks resting on the heels, which are off the ground.

2. Place the fingertips on the floor between the spread knees.

3. Inhale and keep the fingertips on the ground. Lean into your hands and push up, straightening your legs. The buttocks will raise in the air, while the head goes down. Try to bring the nose as close to the knees as possible.

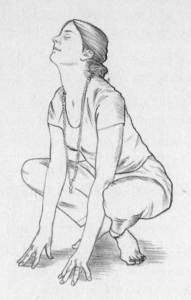 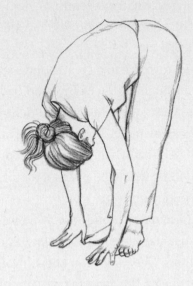

4.  Exhale, come back down, letting the buttocks strike the heels. The inhale and exhale should be powerful.

5.  Start off with eleven frogs at a time, and build up to twenty-six, fifty-four, and eventually one hundred and eight frogs.

As a basic requirement of a healthy individual, we should be in a position to do one hundred and eight frogs at one time. Try to make it a goal to build up to this gradually. As you work up to this, you will find your health improving, physically as well as mentally.

*Effects*: This posture is very rejuvenating, physically and mentally. It can pull all the toxins out of the muscles of the body, especially breaking up blockages in the thighs. This posture helps to channel the sexual energy from the lower triangle to the higher centers; it can also help to straighten out your mind in just a couple of minutes. You will feel the spine getting a good stretch, helping to realign the vertebrae, as well as relaxing back tension.

## SAT KRIYA

For channeling second chakra energy to divinity.

1.    Sit on your heels and stretch the arms over the head, keeping the elbows straight.

2.    Interlock the hands, extending the index fingers so they are pointing straight up.

3.    Begin chanting the mantra "Sat" as you pull in slightly on the rectum, sex organs, and navel point, pulling the energy up from the earth.

4.    Chant "Nam" as you release the locks, and feel the energy go out the top of your head.

5.    The "Sat" is chanted from the navel and is a shorter, more powerful and emphatic sound. "Nam" is more prolonged, relaxed, and releasing.

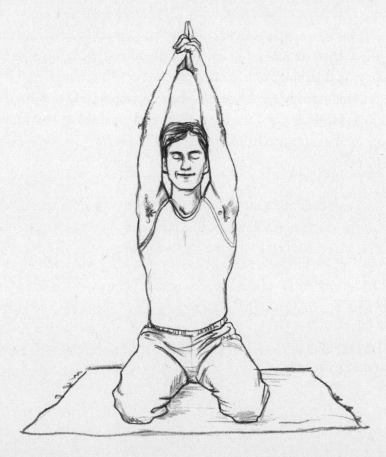

6. Continue for at least three minutes, and then inhale as you pull tightly in on all of the lower locks. Feel the energy moving up your spine, and out the top of your head.

7. Exhale, hold the breath out about ten seconds, squeezing the energy up the spine as you once again pull in on the locks.

8. Then come down and relax on your back.

Ideally you should rest flat on the back in "dead man's pose" for twice as long as you practice Sat Kriya.

9. If you are pregnant or in the first three days of your period, simply come into the posture and softly recite the words without pulling in on the locks.

*Effects:* This is a very basic part of any Kundalini Yoga practice, and can be done on its own or as part of a set. It strengthens the entire sexual system and helps one to direct the sexual energy of the second chakra into your own creativity and healing. Your general physical health is improved, since all the internal organs receive a gentle, rhythmic massage from this exercise. Sat Kriya works directly on stimulating and channeling the Kundalini energy, so it must always be practiced with the mantra, "Sat Nam" (Truth is my Identity).

You can build the time of this *kriya* to thirty-one minutes, but always have a deep relaxation afterwards. It is not just a physical exercise. It works on all levels of your being—known and unknown.

# 3
# The Third Chakra

COMMITMENT

"The pure power of Infinity is in your navel point. You can't buy it, you can't sell it and I cannot give it to you. But I can give you a technological knowledge so that you can initiate it, so it will start working for you in your life."

—Yogi Bhajan

The human talent of commitment is located in the third chakra, what is generally referred to in yogic science as the navel center. It is just below the heart center, encompasses the entire digestive system of the body, and is associated with the liver, the pancreas, the kidneys, and the adrenals. The bull's-eye is the belly button.

We first receive nourishment through this center via the umbilical cord when we are in the womb. This center continues to be a strong source of energy and can make us feel more vibrant and alive when it is activated.

**"Without the activity of the third chakra, a person lives as if in a dungeon. Life means nothing."**

**—Yogi Bhajan**

A person with a well-developed third chakra is usually energetic, organized, and goal-oriented with a powerful projection. Once the third chakra is activated, one does not have to speak to get a message across— generally that person's presence will speak very loudly on its own. Along with this comes a well-developed sense of willpower, commitment, much personal strength, and stamina.

Balance is found when this center is active, because when life is dull and meaningless, we tend to substitute emotions, traumas, and problems to "spice things up." We tend to let things happen to us, rather than direct our choices in life, manifesting our own desires and will.

Someone with an underdeveloped navel point is likely to be seen as scattered, unfocused, without the energy to manifest his thoughts into reality, and consequently frustrated or angry with life and what it has to offer. Common slang tells us a lot about the attributes we already instinctively know to be part of this power center. If someone is very strong in their third chakra we might say, "She's got guts," or "He has a real fire in the belly."

Since this chakra is ruled by the element of fire, it's not surprising that it is associated with the color yellow, the color of the tip of a candle flame. The colors of the first three chakras are red, orange, and yellow. I love the image this gives us; it is just as though these first three power centers of our body form the flame that ignites us into being. In yogic science it is said that the first two power centers are the fuel behind the flame, which gets activated at the third chakra into a strong, directed course of action.

**"Once your third chakra is activated, I am not saying you will have no problems. But you can sit like a lotus in the muddy waters and enjoy life. That is the power of the third chakra. It gives you an instant, infinite experience of your life."**

**—Yogi Bhajan**

A person with a strong navel center has control over his actions, and it is said that the fire of the navel can be used to purify and burn away old patterns of behavior, old habits. Someone who is trying to quit smoking, or who wants to go on a diet, would do well to work on stimulating the third chakra energy and bringing it more fully into his life.

**The first three chakras are like the roots of a tree or the foundation of a building; they are the very base of our physical, as well as energetic, form.**

Traditionally, these first three chakras constitute the lower triangle, and the fifth, sixth, and seventh form the upper triangle. The eight power centers are like floors of a building. No single floor can ever be more valuable than the others. We tend to forget that there is no towering oak without the vast network of roots below.

Another traditional image in the study of the chakras is that of the lotus flower, which has long roots that go down deep into the mud, all to support the delicate blossom at the top. Even with that image there comes judgment; everybody is happy to have a picture of a lotus blossom on their wall, people don't usually want to frame the roots and the muck. It is important that we see the beauty in the foundation, the roots of our system.

When you explore your third chakra and your human talent of commitment, you begin to discover that commitment is the willingness to "be here now." True commitment is to do more for the sake of doing, and not only for the results. Yoga can be experienced fully *as it is happening*, just like life. That's why I always tell students not to quit, no matter what. Even in the hardest, darkest of times, this technology will help you through, and victory will be yours.

**"Your grit is not based on your muscles. Your grit is based on how deeply you breathe. The length and depth of your breath and your sustenance are proportionate."**

**—Yogi Bhajan**

Another interesting function of the navel center chakra is its involvement with respiration, which is primarily a heart chakra function. Although the lungs are in the heart center area, the diaphragm, the muscle that sits below the lungs, is really in the navel center area.

When I was a young girl, we were taught that correct posture involved standing stick-straight and keeping your whole stomach area very firm and tight. As a result, most people of my generation have spent a good part of their lives as shallow lung breathers, which is very unhealthy and leads to medical problems.

As children we went to etiquette school, where we were taught to balance a book on our heads as we walked, holding in our stomachs. Later, when I was a cheerleader in high school, we were constantly instructed to suck in our stomachs. I remember my favorite cousin, who was older than I, and who became one of the first airline stewardesses in history, which was a very big deal in the fifties. She would drill my sister and me in posture, emphatically insisting that we hold in our stomachs as far as possible. Repeatedly I was instructed to hold in my stomach and not to breathe. That's just how it was if you were a girl growing up when I did.

**If you only take one thing away from this entire book let it be this: Stop holding your breath, and begin breathing from your abdominals.**

**"The length and depth of your breath measures the effect of your psyche on the other person's psyche. What makes you attractive to another person is how deeply and slowly you breathe. There was a time when there were special schools and monasteries for this kind of training."**

**—Yogi Bhajan**

Let's go over what will happen if you do as I suggest. If you totally let your stomach muscles relax as you inhale, your diaphragm will open, and your lungs will fill to their full capacity, maybe for the first time in years. *Now* you are breathing as God intended you to breathe.

### EXERCISE
### LEARNING TO BREATHE

1.  Stand erect.
2.  Open a hardcover book as if you are reading it, and press the lower edges against your navel.
3.  As you inhale, your belly pushes the book away from your body.
4.  As you exhale, the book glides back towards the spine, as the belly empties.
5.  Continue for three minutes.

As you inhale, you fill up that belly cavity, allowing the breath to circulate fully through your bloodstream. At this point, your blood will become more highly oxygenated, which will fuel all your organs, most specifically all the nerve cells in your brain, and you will begin to think more clearly.

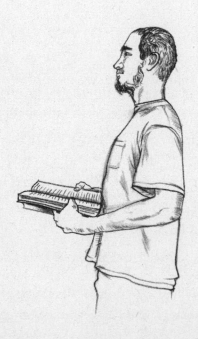

**Breathe right; it's your birthright.**

And what does all of this have to do with the human talent of commitment? Only everything, that's all. Because if you can commit to your breath, you can commit to anything. In every movie I've ever seen, when the hero or heroine had to do something requiring real commitment, like jumping off a moving train, the first thing they always did was to take a deep breath.

You might find if you make a really conscious effort to breathe in this way, you may want to make certain changes. Foremost among these is not wearing clothing that is too restricting. Dress however it pleases you, but if your clothing is too tight and restricts your breathing, you might want to reconsider your priorities. I have students who cripple their breathing because they are unwilling to admit that the size of jeans they wear may have changed since they were fifteen. I guarantee you that the extra oxygen will do more to enhance your health and life than a certain number at your waistband.

> **"Your entire way of life can change if you change your clothing and your food."**
>
> **—Yogi Bhajan**

If you decide to make breath a priority, more often than not you will find your pants size dropping anyway, almost as if by magic. People who really make a commitment to their breath, in my experience, seem to be less ruled by food cravings. It's almost as if by allowing your third chakra to function naturally, your stomach stops sending you false messages of hunger. Most of the time, you are probably more hungry for breath than you are for food. There are legends of yogis who live off the breath. They are called "breatharians."

**It's amazing what acceptance can do, even for a body part.**

I'm not saying you will have massive weight loss through breath alone. I will say that I have seen massive weight loss among my long-term students. Moreover, I see almost no obesity among those who take up a reasonable schedule of yoga, doing it only twice a week. I don't scientifically monitor my students. I don't know what else they are doing, I only know what I observe. People who commit to doing even a moderate amount of yoga over the long term seem to have consistent and healthy body weights. Not the false fashion industry ideal of the super-model, but healthy, active, strong bodies that can move. When you breathe consciously, your food choices naturally change. You will probably find yourself eating more fresh fruits and vegetables. This will make you feel better, because you will be relating to the life force of the universe. With every exhale, you are giving back to the earth to grow these fruits and vegetables.

Almost more than any other body part, people seem to have distorted images of the stomach area.

I recently saw an episode of the television show *48 Hours* that featured a young man who was anorexic because he believed that he had a "fat stomach." This man spent hours in the gym, working only this area of his body, sure that he was repulsive to all. In the paradox that is anorexia, he was repulsive to people because of his emaciated frame. He eventually overcame this extreme view of his own body, but I wonder how many of us harbor a less extreme but equally distorted vision of ourselves?

For good health our bellies should extend slightly beyond our hip bones, as opposed to the fashionable ideal. Commit to allowing yourself to accept your stomach and your third chakra area.

I once had a student who was plagued with chronic middle back problems. He had breathed incorrectly all his life, and often had such severe seizures of the middle back that he was bedridden. He was in his late thirties at this point, and had been to many chiropractors. Back surgery had even been suggested when this student finally found his way to Golden Bridge as a last-ditch effort to avoid going under the knife.

I worked with him one-on-one, and confirmed what I believed to be true: This student held his stomach muscles rigidly and almost never inhaled or exhaled a complete breath as a result. I showed him the correct way to breathe, which unlike improper breath takes almost no "work"—only awareness and commitment. Incorrect breathing involves people lifting up their entire rib cage and hunching their shoulders, squeezing their bellies on the inhale, which is, of course, a tremendous amount of effort as compared to simply letting your belly relax out, rise up, and then lower again on the exhale.

I challenged this student to spend an entire day focused on his breath. We talked about what it would entail, and he made a firm commitment to do it. He chose a Saturday, when he would be more relaxed and not involved in his usual high-pressure job. He worked in the health care profession, spending his days caring for others, but he was unable to care for himself in the most basic way, by simply getting his lungs full of good fresh air.

**A shadow emotion of the third chakra is anger.**

My student told me that by lunchtime of "Breathing Day" he was almost ready to give up. He found it very difficult, and found himself getting more and more angry. I had anticipated that it would bring up a lot of anger in him, and had warned him this would happen. When the third chakra is insufficient, a person has to compensate for it. Consequently, it may not come as a surprise to you to know anger as the shadow emotion of the third chakra.

Once again, if you look to cliches and aphorisms you see that folk wisdom recognizes that anger lives primarily in our third chakra. When we refer to someone who is too angry, we might say they are "full of bile." Bile is a substance produced by the liver, which is located in the third chakra. If we are angry at someone we might say, "He makes me sick to my stomach," or "She makes me want to puke."

So back to the student who couldn't breathe. He decided to stick with his "Breathing Day" despite the anger he was feeling. He focused on breathing as he had learned, right up until he went to bed, despite his anger and annoyance. Since he had made the commitment to see it through, just for that one day, he stuck it out. He felt a kind of victory as he went to bed that night, and then he slept for twelve hours straight. He told me it was the most fantastic sleep he had ever experienced, and he felt great the next day.

He was so amazed by the way that he had slept, he made a conscious effort to continue this way of breathing the next day as well. The results weren't as dramatic, but he wasn't as angered by this "belly breath" either.

Gradually, he began to breathe this way all the time, but it took conscious awareness. He says it still takes effort. He has to focus on his breath consciously some days, especially when he is feeling angry or stressed out. As he told me, "It's worth it to pay attention to my breath because I feel so much better. There are some things worth paying attention to and this is one of them. If I'm driving on the freeway, I have to pay attention, or I'll have an accident. That's just logical. Paying attention to my breath is similar, although I have a slightly wider margin of error." Certainly it's true, falling into your old bad breathing pattern won't likely get you hit by a semi. But unhealthy breathing could be just as dangerous, since it is a contributing factor to many, many diseases.

"Evolved human beings have very calm breath. Normally you breathe fifteen times a minute. If you breathe ten times a minute you'll be very energetic. If you breathe five times a minute you'll be very intelligent. If you can breathe one time a minute you will become invincible. The power of the breath should be under your own control."

—Yogi Bhajan

The health benefits for this student of changing his breathing pattern have been phenomenal. By doing nothing more than a fairly regular practice of yoga and this conscious breath, he has had a complete cessation of his chronic back problems, and there has been no more talk of surgery.

In working with this student, I wondered how he might have become this dysfunctional in his breathing. I was saddened to discover that he had deep patterns of anger in his life, running to his early childhood. He had a father who abandoned him and his siblings at a very young age, and a physically abusive mother.

I had always seen a lot of anger in this young man. When I first met him, he would often complain about what I was asking the class to do. He would always say that a certain exercise was "impossible." Naturally, he had also said that breathing from your navel, which is what I call breathing from your diaphragm, was impossible. It was as if this word, "impossible," was the flash point for anything and everything he felt angry about in his life.

Granted, this student had reason to be angry, more than most of us, but that was never what really seemed to anger him. All the mundane annoyances of life, like bad traffic and broken appliances and a difficult yoga exercise, seemed to be the focus of his rage and anger. It wasn't the core issue of his abusive childhood, it was the stupid clerk at the post office who was making him angry, and making life itself "impossible."

When we are in the womb, we imprint many physical and emotional patterns from our mothers. We learn the breathing patterns of our mother. Some of our mothers smoked, drank, or were full of rage and fear. Some were encouraged to be sedated into unconsciousness during our births. When we were born, our breath came naturally, but as we grew older, we began to imitate the respiration we felt all those months in the womb. We return to the patterning given to us by our mothers.

This student, like all of us, had patterns of behavior to heal, all the way down to his breath. He had been studying Kundalini Yoga and Meditation for a few years before he began his commitment to conscious breathing. Around this same time, he got into a support group and began to acknowledge the feelings of anger he had toward both his parents, and further healing happened. Today I see him as a greatly changed person. The constant furrow between his brows has disappeared, and his true, sensitive nature is beginning to emerge from the obscuring clutter of his ever-present anger.

I became aware of just how much this student had grown when I saw him in class one day. He was sitting far in the back of the class as he always does, but I noticed he was wearing a T-shirt that had the word "Impossible" on it. It gave me a little laugh, because I knew that he still got frustrated with certain exercises, but I wasn't hearing him say that things seemed impossible anymore. He usually just did his best. I thought that maybe the T-shirt was just a remnant of his old attitude, a wry little joke on himself.

After class, when we gathered for tea and cookies, I got quite a surprise. I went over to give him a hug and noticed that the shirt didn't say "Impossible"—it said, "I'm possible." We both had a good laugh. He said he wears it to remind himself how he used to think and feel, and how different that is from how he thinks and feels now. When I asked him what he thought the most important tool in his growth had been, he replied, "Without a doubt, it was the breath. Learning to breathe from my belly has changed my life." Not so impossible after all.

**Anyone who makes even the smallest effort to heal himself is taking an enormous step towards becoming alive. I admire everyone who practices Kundalini Yoga and Meditation.**

Emotions can be used for positive goals or negative ones. If you can remember to turn your emotion into devotion, you will know what to do with potentially destructive emotions like anger.

When I think of fearlessness and commitment, so many of my students come to mind.

I feel very privileged that I get to see people after they have already made the decision to do something positive about their lives. It's one of the great blessings of my life.

Sometimes, in my everyday life, I come across people who seem to come out of nowhere, who touch me because they are so gifted and full of grace. A few months back, as I was taking a walk in my little neighborhood here in L.A., I met a woman who touched me deeply because of her level of commitment.

She was an ancient, elfin little person, walking in front of me, pushing a shopping cart. I assumed she might be a homeless person, in her tattered, faded, red coat. As I got closer, I noticed that her shopping cart was full of bags of bread. One of the wheels was sticking, and she was having a hard time crossing the street, so I bent down to help her, and together we made it safely across.

When we got to the other side, I was rewarded with effusive thanks and a smile that seemed luminous even in the arid L.A. sunshine. She was cheerful, and struck up a conversation almost instantly. I fancied myself to be in a hurry, but didn't want to be impolite, so I listened to what she was telling me.

She didn't live in this neighborhood, and everyone here knew her as the "Bird Lady." Every day she took three buses to get to my neighborhood, where there is a very nice city park. Once she arrived, she would make the rounds of all the local bakeries, getting day-old baked goods, which she would carry in a shopping cart to the park. There, she would feed an enormous flock of pigeons that waited for her. She never missed a day; she was always there, and the birds always waited. She said sometimes even the seagulls came all the way from the ocean to eat her bread. She seemed to know all the birds.

I thought it was sweet to devote her life to feeding a flock of birds. Certainly she was committed, but what value did this commitment have in the larger scope of the world? She intrigued me, so I decided to join her on her journey the next day, and that is when I learned something remarkable. When we commit to something, anything that is basically good, no matter how small, it has a huge effect on other people, in ways that are almost impossible to quantify.

I went with her to the local bakeries, where she was cheerfully greeted by each of the owners. They were happy to see her and happy to do something besides throw away what was perfectly good food. I sat with her in the park. Many of the local children and adults in that park would come by and feed the birds alongside her.

Everyone who strolled by ostensibly came to join her in feeding the birds, but I noticed that she knew a lot about all the people who stopped, and was a gifted and eager listener. A child updated her on a project she was working on for school; a young weary mom told her about her difficult nights with a colicky baby; a cop who walks the beat in the park told her about problems he was having with a young boy he mentors. To each of these people she offered a kind ear and her sweet mischievous little smile, along with another handful of crumbs.

She would inevitably murmur some words of encouragement, nothing huge or profound, but everything she said was received eagerly and gratefully. As people went on their way, they seemed relieved, somehow restored, just from the five minutes or so they had spent with the Bird Lady.

In this way she seemed to function as the elder wise woman of the neighborhood. There were so many people whose lives she obviously touched on a daily basis. She wasn't appointed by any commission, she didn't receive a grant, she just made a simple commitment, and put her whole self into what she had committed to do. She would be there every day to feed the birds, and in the process she also fed many humans spiritually.

I asked her how many years she had been doing this. She said she started in Rumania. She came to America in her fifties. She has been feeding the birds every day since she came to this country, almost fifty years.

As I spent those few hours with her, I became deeply aware of how some people really function almost as angels in our lives, and how by her attitude and her commitment, this woman brought healing and hope to so many people in my little neighborhood.

The lesson I learned from the Bird Lady is that you don't have to do anything earthshaking to make a real difference in people's lives, you just have to be present, committed to whatever it is you do. You can be of service in the most mundane way, if you are present and committed every moment of the day. The Bird Lady was a master of this. She is forever with me in my heart.

In fact, this story of the Bird Lady reminds me of an old Zen fable I heard once. There was a traveling Zen master who was wandering in the countryside of Japan, followed by a handful of his devoted students who were very proud of him. As they traveled through a small village, they attracted the attention of a Buddhist monk who followed a different teacher.

This Buddhist monk wondered what it was about the traveling Zen master that inspired such devotion. The monk stopped one of the Zen master's students and said to him, "I also follow a master, and he is a very powerful and magical man. He can wave his arm in the air, writing letters in the sky. If someone is standing nearby with a piece of paper in their hand, the characters magically appear on that sheet of paper. Can your master do any feats as great as that?"

The student of the traveling Zen master thought for a moment and then replied, "My master is very magical, too. When he sits down to eat, he eats. When he walks, he walks. And when he talks, he talks."

The inquiring monk thought about this. Humbled, he then said, "Your master is a very gifted man. I think I will follow him too so that one day when I am walking, I too will simply walk."

I love that story, because to be able to commit to seeing every day as a brand new day is the human challenge. My new friend, the Bird Lady, was just such a master, and I'm thankful I didn't rush past her, too busy to learn the valuable lesson she had to offer me.

**Yoga and meditation are a lifelong practice that can help remind us of how exactly to "be here, now."**

EXERCISE

STRETCH POSE

Perhaps the most powerful exercise in all of Kundalini Yoga is the very ineptly named "stretch pose." The name implies that this exercise is some sort of long, languorous, delicious stretch, but this pose is anything *but* that. It is unbelievably challenging, and no matter how many times you do it, you will most likely always find it to be a challenge.

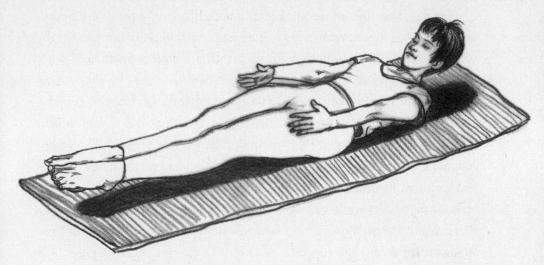

I realize that I am not giving it a great buildup, and you may be think-ing, "No way," or "Why bother?" But here is the other side of stretch pose, the sweet benefit. If you try it, even for a few seconds, quit, and then keep trying, even for as little as one minute total, you will be changed on some level. And the more you succeed at it, the more your human talent of com-mitment will be enriched. Absolutely guaranteed.

Although the pose is difficult for almost everyone, it is doable by almost everyone.

1.  Lie flat on your back on something soft but firm.
2.  Raise your head, hands, and heels six inches off the ground, press-ing your chin into your chest. Lift your shoulders off the ground, but keep the shoulder blades pressed into the ground.
3.  Stretch your hands towards your pointed toes.
4.  Stare at your big toes.
5.  Begin breath of fire through your nose.

Breath of fire is a very rapid inhalation and exhalation through your nostrils. Remember the dog breath we did in one of our last exercises? It's similar to that, only it's done through your nose instead of through the open mouth. You breathe by pumping your navel like a bellows—as you inhale the belly goes out, and as you exhale the belly goes in. You can even watch your belly as you are staring at your toes, if you want.

Breath of fire is the most powerful breath. It totally strengthens your nervous system, purifies your blood, energizes you, and makes you feel better and brighter. Doing breath of fire in stretch pose can actually help you keep up in the posture!

In stretch pose, if your lower back needs support, you can place your hands under your buttocks, palms down, and do the above. If your neck needs support, you can place a hand under the back of the neck. Lastly, if you are in the first three days of your menstrual cycle, or your lower back needs something more gentle, raise one leg at a time and hold for thirty seconds on each side, while you do long deep breathing through your nose. Remember to keep staring at your toes! Do not do stretch pose at all if you are pregnant!

6. After completing one to three minutes of stretch pose, totally relax into corpse pose.

If you do a difficult pose and your body starts shaking, I say welcome the shaking. It's better to shake a little now as you heal your nervous system, than to shake when you are old, and not be able to stop.

In about two seconds you will see why I say it is challenging. You might start to shake a little as you do this. Many students are afraid of this shaking when it first occurs, but I always tell them to welcome it. The seventy-two thousand nerve endings, which yogic science describes as meeting at your navel point, are being energized, and are beginning to repair themselves. The shaking is a good thing. With yoga, we release a lot of energy that was previously stored in our muscles as tension. When this energy suddenly surges through us, it can be quite a shock to our nervous system, but in reality the weak or broken connections between the nerves are being reestablished. You may shake a little, but as your nerves get stronger and can take the higher voltage, the shaking will stop. After doing stretch pose daily, you will stop shaking and start to feel very strong and centered.

Do it for one minute, and work up to three minutes every morning. If you have to keep going in and out of the pose, that's fine. Many students who have studied for years still end up going in and out of this pose when we do it in class. All that matters is that you make the commitment to lift your head and legs up after you have set them down. If you can only hold the pose for a few seconds at a time, that's great; that's a victory. Focus on your breath. Really listen to your breath, feel your breath, and stare at your toes.

Stretch pose puts everyone through a lot. You will get emotional doing stretch pose. You may cry or get angry and possibly have emotional outbursts toward anyone and everyone who comes to mind. That's fine, that's why we do stretch pose. Whatever you are feeling was already there before you began the exercise. Kundalini Yoga simply brings it to the surface and creates a healing. Plus, it allows you to go beyond your limits, expanding your horizons.

> **Use your yoga practice to feel your emotions on a physical level; then as you experience them, you can move past them and become victorious over them.**

> **"Emotions are like guests. They should be treated very nicely and gently, and sent away if they don't fit in."**
> **—Yogi Bhajan**

Stretch pose will strengthen your commitment. Commitment is stronger and more powerful than any shadow emotions. Once again, a simple physical posture expands you spiritually and mentally, using the vehicle of your human body as the means for this growth.

If anger is coming dangerously close to getting the best of you, do this posture for one to three minutes. You will be able to channel all that energy and emotion into something more constructive. You will be able to use that fire in the belly as a roaring fire in a fireplace, instead of burning down the whole house. You will know, almost on a cellular level, that as a human being, you do not have to give in to your emotions. Stretch pose can be a powerful tool in letting this fire energy be used constructively.

**Anger can rule your life only if you let it.**

If you need to control your anger, and doing stretch pose is not a practical option, there is a very simple breathing meditation that will help you to "cool down."

### COOL-DOWN MEDITATION: SITALI PRANAYAM

There is a wonderful breathing meditation I was taught by my beloved teacher, Yogi Bhajan, for any time you need to get in touch with your own regenerative powers, and pull yourself out of a negative state of mind.

1. Stick your tongue out slightly, and if you can, curl it upward into a tube shape. Most people can do this, but some people find it impossible. It's a matter of genetics for the most part. So, stick your tongue out, curl it to the best of your ability, and think of using it like a straw.

2. You are going to breathe in through your mouth, using the straw of your tongue to draw in the breath, and then expel it completely, through the nose. The breath is powerful, long, and deep.

3. Keep your eyes closed and focused at your third eye point.

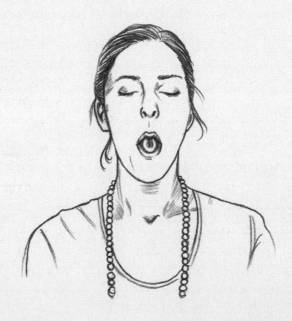

Try the breath pattern at first for three minutes. You can just set a clock or timer in front of you, and open your eyes when you want to take a peek at how much time has elapsed. After you do it for a while, you may find you actually begin to crave doing it for a longer period because it is so rejuvenating. Start with three minutes, then maybe try seven, eleven, twenty-six, or even thirty-one.

*Effects:* This breathing meditation is very simple, but it may put you through a lot of changes. It is very strengthening and cleansing, and you may begin to sense a slight metallic taste in your mouth. This is simply the result of toxins that are being excreted through the breath and mouth. The bad taste will go away after a while, and you will begin tasting sweetness. According to ancient yogic science, it is when you taste this sweetness that you will know that the rejuvenating powers of the body are becoming active.

I find this meditation to be amazing because even after a few rounds, I feel noticeably better. This meditation can be practiced for twenty-six times in the morning and twenty-six times in the evening. The ancient yogis say doing fifty-two breaths daily can extend your life span. It is the breath that is immediately turned to whenever anyone is sick and has a fever, because it has such a cooling effect.

During this exercise you may find the body getting itchy. This is because the nerves, liver, and spleen are all being adjusted. As a result, the nerves are making a new connection, which sometimes causes a lot of muscle twitching. Just stay steady and go through it.

Whenever you need stamina, power, and strength, therein lies the secret of the *sitali pranayam*. It helps rid the psyche of fear, disease, sickness—all sorts of nonsense that we go through. And just think, the cure is right inside of you!

This is a terrific meditation to teach a small child. You can play it as a game, so it can be something the child may try on his own, when he feels scared or overwhelmed by his feelings. A number of parents are using it, and find that it works.

I should mention here that children really enjoy most yoga postures and meditations. Because of their natural flexibility, they are bound to find some postures much easier than most adults. I find that it's fun for them to do what the adults are trying to do, and be able to do it better.

Every Thanksgiving, I have a big waffle brunch. We always have a giant yoga class beforehand to which the students bring their whole families—kids, grandparents, et cetera. The kids, even the tiniest of infants, always seem to be delighted by the fact that the adults are stretching and bending their bodies, which is of course something infants do all day long. If you really want to let your children experience a feeling of success, teach them a yoga pose you have been trying, and then give them lots of praise when they automatically do it perfectly, as they inevitably will.

The whistle breath is one of the simplest ways to defuse that feeling of uncontrollable anger. The image of it, as though we were literally a little tea kettle blowing off steam, is very soothing to me. If you find that you like this meditation in a one- or three-minute session, you will find it deeply relaxing if you do it for a seven- or eleven-minute period. It's definitely one of those meditations that can make you feel almost "high." This whistle breath can have a calming effect on many unsettling emotions.

**Repressed anger will express itself through disease.**

Domestic violence, including verbal abuse, is prevalent in so many families. It happens in mansions, and it happens in slums, it just seems to happen everywhere. There seems to be so much free-floating anger that has no where to go.

Certainly, there are many reasons for this, but anger is something that has to be dealt with on an individual basis. No one can remove someone else's anger. The only thing that works is to focus on your own anger. If you are with someone who is chronically and toxically angry, there is no course of behavior you can adopt that will ever reduce that person's anger. If you are dealing with someone else's anger on a chronic basis, you are building up a huge amount of corresponding anger response of your own.

**If you do not acknowledge your repressed anger, this emotion may express itself through the form of disease, for example, cancer.**

For a time, so-called primal scream therapy was in vogue. Theoretically, if you used verbalization, you'd be able to "vent" your anger, process it, and then get rid of it. Studies have shown that screaming and yelling actually do nothing to reduce anger, and can in fact increase the levels of stressor neurotransmitters in people's bloodstream, only increasing their anxiety. A study done at Duke University bore out the idea that people who verbally express anger have a higher early mortality rate than those who don't. Yoga and meditation are a way to channel this anger to construct, rather than destroy, your life.

Although Western medical science has recently acknowledged that stress has a major impact on our health, only very recently has research begun to separate out various emotions and study their specific effects on our health and well-being. Dr. Redford Williams has written a wonderful book entitled *Anger Kills*, in which he details the very specific health effects of verbally expressed anger. Based on clinical studies he has done, he has discovered that patients, especially men, can literally kill themselves with their own anger. According to Dr. Williams, "Those with high hostility levels are four to seven times more likely to be dead of coronary disease and other causes by age fifty."

My father was a perfect example of this. He was born in 1894. He died when I was nineteen years old, back in the early sixties. When I was growing up, there were no self-help tools we could use to help us through life's problems. We didn't talk about alcoholism, we just talked about "Old Harry, the drunk down the street." If a person was full of rage, we apologized for him, saying, "Oh, that's just George, he's got a hot head."

No one understood the relationship of our emotional patterning and our physical health. As a result, my father basically died of anger and rage, because he had no way to deal with those emotions, no place to put them, no tools to heal. He couldn't channel them in useful ways, and ultimately those emotions killed him. Bless his soul.

When we express verbal anger, it has a detrimental health outcome on those around us, but as Dr. Williams's research clearly shows, it has an effect on us as well. If your reaction is just to "put up and shut up," you are still going to be in trouble, because there are serious health consequences to this plan of action. Another study, this one done by the American Psychological Association, found a direct link between smoking addiction in women and anger. In the study, the angrier the women were, the more they smoked.

I smoked in my younger years, along with using speed and caffeine. I, too, was full of rage. I took on the patterning of my dominant parent, my father. A therapist told me once that I wasn't angry. I felt proud of myself at that moment, until he continued, "No, you're not angry, in fact, you're full of rage." It took a lot for me to be able to accept that. I had to stop denying that I had taken on the emotional pattern of my father. When I accepted that, I was able to seek help in healing. I finally understood that happiness was my birthright.

The whole issue of anger is a catch-22. If I express anger, it's bad for me, and if I don't, it's bad for me. Kundalini Yoga and Meditation provide us with a way out of this cycle. I don't think it's the only answer; certainly therapy and other techniques are beneficial as well, and I always encourage any student to use every tool that's available. You can do Kundalini Yoga and Meditation for yourself right away, it costs so little, and it will open up the doors to a world of healing possibilities.

Let's examine the way yogic science takes a look at this issue of anger. According to yogic philosophy, the primary place anger begins to manifest in the body is in the liver. The liver is an amazing endocrine gland, literally an ingenious filtering system, designed to remove poisons from our bloodstream. The liver is an organ that will put up with a lot before it begins to cause us trouble. We all know that cirrhosis of the liver is often caused by alcoholism or drug abuse, and usually occurs after we put what are essentially poisons into our body for many years. Eventually, the liver just can't handle the constant work and begins to shut down.

**The most basic commitment any human can make is the commitment to being fully alive.** ← wow!

Most of my life as a yoga teacher has been spent working with people who are trying to overcome chemical dependency. One thing I hear over and over is that people drink or use drugs because they don't know where to put their rage. Not knowing what to do, and fearful of telling anyone, they slip into the darkness of addiction.

If you abuse alcohol or drugs, you cannot ever say yes to life. Some people may argue that you don't know it's poison, but anyone who has ever had even one hangover knows that what got him there was poison. People may deny it, but they know it. Physically, you can just feel it. When you detox, the pain and aggravation you feel tells you this.

There are many people who manage to destroy their liver without substances. I had a student—again, someone who had settled for a very high-pressure job she hated. On the recommendation of a doctor with whom I work, she came to me because her liver was malfunctioning. She was only twenty-five years old, and yet she was so miserable that the doctor had originally thought she had hepatitis. What he discovered was her liver had begun to malfunction strictly because of the catchall phrase, "job stress."

When he spoke to her more extensively about her job situation, he began to see it was really her stuffed anger at not doing work she enjoyed that was making her so stressed out. It wasn't the work itself that was highly stressful; it was simply the wrong work for her. She felt she was wasting her life by doing it. In this young woman's case, any job that wasn't at least heading her toward her dream would have been a high-stress job. As she puts it, "They could have been paying me a million bucks a day to take naps, and I still would have been a wreck."

She began doing Kundalini Yoga, and this led her, like so many students, to make different choices about her work. She has made some changes, committed to living on less money, and has gone back to school to study what she really enjoys. By the way, her liver is now functioning perfectly.

This student also took a couple of dietary recommendations from me. I don't often make them, because there are a lot of people who are more knowledgeable about nutrition than I am. When it comes to the liver, there are two things I can enthusiastically recommend. The first is to eat as many beets and beet greens as you possibly can. If you drink beet juice, drink only two ounces per day. The second recommendation is to eat radishes of any kind, but particularly Japanese daikon radishes. Both are real "super-foods" when it comes to healing the liver. And, of course, yogi tea is also a great and tasty way to flush the liver.

I helped direct a drug and rehab center some years ago in Tucson, Arizona. We had one of the highest rates of recovery in the U.S. The modality was Kundalini Yoga, meditation, diet, massage, and hydrotherapy. In my extensive work with people in recovery, I see what a difference including these foods in the diet can make in the whole liver detox process.

## ADRENALS

The other main gland that we find in the third chakra, the adrenals, also play a role in what I call the "anger-stress cycle."

The adrenals are remarkable glands, producing adrenaline and cortisol, which your body uses to physically prime itself for response to any kind of "fight or flight" situation it encounters.

This system worked well when most of the stresses we encountered in our daily lives were physical threats, requiring a physical response. This system was perfect when the stressful situation we encountered was a big tiger up ahead! Adrenaline and cortisol primed us to run. For most people, the stress they encounter today is not a tiger, but a demanding boss, or an irritated customer, or an angry husband. Our poor endocrine system keeps pumping out those hormones and neuropeptides just as if we were being chased by a tiger. What gets left out of this cycle is the fact that when the tiger chased us we would run, and these very powerful hormones and neuropeptides would be burned out of our systems through physical exertion.

Kundalini Yoga, which focuses most specifically on glandular health and rejuvenation, is a discipline that can save us from the killing effect of this stress-anger cycle. Thousands of studies tell us that stress and anger have a detrimental effect on our health, and exercise is often cited as a way to combat this. Most exercises are designed just to strengthen a particular muscle; they are generally not expected to have a beneficial effect on glands or organs. Often the approach to exercise you find in many health clubs is so relentlessly focused on physical appearance that it seems to produce a stress-anger cycle all its own.

Kundalini Yoga works on glandular and organ systems. Countless students have healed themselves of a specific problem by doing a practice of Kundalini Yoga for the chakras that were most involved with their condition. I see the most improvement in students who focus on the specific meditation and yoga that will help them in their life situations. These are the students who commit themselves to awareness, who believe they can develop and grow. If a student will commit to doing an exercise or meditation for forty days, the miracles begin to occur, because it takes that length of time for re-patterning to begin.

I have seen the most improvement in those students who didn't just merely focus on a chakra, but on the imbalances they had in that chakra. Those students who took this extra step were always the cases for whom the most miraculous healing occurred.

And the human talents have a domino effect on each other as well. For example, when we are committed to a practice of Kundalini Yoga and Meditation, we begin to feel more gratitude for a body that is beginning to function at a higher level of efficiency. Consequently, when our bodies aren't constantly besieged by disease, we become even more grateful, and have more time to love our lives. Living in truth begins to make us aware of the greater truths of the universe, which we receive through our intuition. In that way, the cycle goes on and on.

**Each human talent resonates up and down on this beautifully interconnected system of chakras.**

When I cast my mind back, thinking of students who focused not just on the physical work but on the deficiency of a specific human talent, I always think of one student. This woman had the most remarkable case of physical recovery I have ever seen.

Now in her early forties, she is a busy executive with an abundance of vitality and an irresistibly infectious laugh. She is physically strong, and if you didn't know her story, you would say she was just a typical physically fit yoga student.

When this woman came to Kundalini Yoga, she came under a doctor's death sentence. She had been told she had six months to live. She had spent her twenties in a very dangerous lifestyle, as a call girl and an exotic dancer. She had been addicted to alcohol and cigarettes and was also an occasional drug user. When I asked her to describe herself at that time, she said, "On the outside I was all about having fun, getting my kicks. I didn't think about the future, and never thought about God or spirituality or anything like that. I just wanted to be cute and have everything I wanted. But inside I was angry, all the time. I had a terrible temper, I used to just go off on people, I was like an explosion just waiting to happen. I drank and used drugs to quiet the anger, but it never worked, not really."

She had given up her life as a sex worker, and had become a successful businesswoman, but that anger still simmered in her. She got involved in a very contentious lawsuit, and it was at a time she started to feel very ill. She lost a lot of weight, couldn't eat, was vomiting all the time. She was prescribed an incredible number of drugs, antidepressants, sleeping pills, diuretics, antifungals, and nothing seemed to work. She was getting sicker all the time.

The doctors finally discovered she had cirrhosis of the liver and hepatitis C, both potentially fatal illnesses, and was told she needed a liver transplant. In an even more devastating blow, she was told not only was she HIV positive, but she had full-blown AIDS. Her T-cell count was 70, while a normal person would have a count of at least 400. Her doctors told her she needed to get her affairs in order, because she had only six months to live.

She had become a Buddhist by this point. She gradually began to accept her own death, but then she made a very radical change in her pattern of behavior. She made a commitment. Her whole life had been about avoiding commitment of any kind, including the commitment to be a fully present, sober human on the planet earth. She decided she would finally make a commitment, the commitment to have a graceful death. To experience life on life's terms, even as she was bidding it farewell.

**Commitment can be your salvation.**

She quit smoking and drinking. She began eating a healthy whole-food, vegetarian diet, understanding and honoring each food she ate. She began walking. She had never exercised and it was very difficult for her. Her first commitment was literally to walk around the block. She did, and it was her first victory. She began walking farther and farther. She says it helps her to connect with God, to know her place in this intricate pattern of existence. She still walks.

One day she walked into a Kundalini Yoga class, because she felt as if she needed something more. She committed to this science of yoga like almost no other student I have ever seen. Commitment can be the beginning of your salvation, and it *was* for this student. Because she was trying so hard to let go of her anger, and heal her liver, she did a set we call "Let the Liver Live."

It's not an easy collection of postures, but she did it twice a day, every day. I asked her what it was that made her, someone who previously couldn't walk around the block, persevere in doing this set. She said, "It's hard to explain, because these exercises are so strange when you look at them objectively, but the fact was, I felt something changing in me. After I did the yoga, I could really feel a change. I began to see an image of my liver becoming healthy, of all the poisonous emotions of anger and hatred being drained away from me. And I also did a lot of heat treatments, because I heard that HIV hates heat, so I began to love heat. I found out that the toxins in the liver are excreted through the skin in sweat, so I began to love to sweat. I began to change my goal from dying well to living fully. I knew that the yoga was healing me, so I kept coming back."

She went to New Mexico in the summer for our women's yoga camp and Summer Solstice Celebration. Back in Los Angeles, she came to every class she could fit into her work schedule and continued doing the yoga on her own, every day. The six-month due date of her death came, and passed, and she was still here.

Her healing had begun with her increasing commitment. There were tangible signs that the poison of her anger and disease was in fact draining out of her body. Her T-cell count started to come up, as did her liver enzymes. She no longer had to get up early enough to finish her vomiting in time to get to work. She now does yoga in what used to be her "morning nausea time," and not surprisingly, she says, "It's way more fun!"

Although she remains on aggressive AIDS medication, she began slowly to wean herself off the dizzying array of prescription medications she had been taking. She cut out the sleeping pills, which gave her the courage to go off the antidepressants, the diuretics, the antifungals, the antibiotics, and the high blood pressure medication.

She did all this under the supervision of her doctor. Her doctor is not someone who believes in any kind of alternative therapies or healing practices, but even he had to acknowledge that her recovery was remarkable, and he now grudgingly admits, "She must be doing something right."

It has been exactly five years since she was told that she had six months to live. Today, she is free of the hepatitis C virus, her liver functions normally, and there has been no more thought of her needing a transplant. The HIV viral load is at zero in her bloodstream and her T-cell count is now over 300. She is confident that as they continue to rise there will come a day when even her skeptical doctor will be forced to admit that she no longer has AIDS.

She has made use of many alternative healing modalities. She takes acupuncture, and uses a variety of vitamins and supplements. She is very open-minded now, and will try almost anything. When I asked her if she considered yoga the main treatment responsible for her healing, she told me that she didn't really think it was important to know what exactly had healed her. She then reminded me of something I had said in class. When you are making ice cream, it is very hard to know just exactly when it ceases to be milk and cream and sugar, and to pinpoint when it definitely becomes ice cream. It's all a process, and it's important to just keep on cranking. Stopping to analyze it certainly isn't going to help make it become ice cream, so why bother?

Today, it is hard to believe that she would once have described herself as "a person who is angry all the time." She is a delight to be around, always the first person to laugh at a good joke, or tell one. Her commitment to her yoga practice has only increased, to the point where she took teacher training, and is now studying an ancient form of yoga meditation called "Sat Nam Rasayan," which involves meditating for the healing of another person.

She continues to work as a businesswoman, but feels called to be a healer. She says that now her life has beauty, meaning, and purpose. She doesn't know how this call will be manifested in her life, she is just intuitively taking steps in educating herself and knowing that God will lead her where she is supposed to be.

I can testify that she is a healer already. Seeing her commitment has healed me, because it reminds me of the awesome power of this work. As I watch her interacting with the other students, I see her as a joy-filled person who brings light into the lives of others.

You may be reading this and thinking, "That's all well and good, but I don't have that kind of time. I don't want to do that much, I just don't." The fact is, you don't have to. If you begin to honor your commitment on even the smallest level, you will see growth and healing in your life. Even if you commit to listening to the boring story someone desperately needs to tell at a party, you will reap a benefit.

**If you commit to doing a yoga exercise or meditation, even for a minute, you will reap a benefit.**

This student healed herself on a grand scale, and other students heal themselves at their own rate and pace. Every one of them is an ongoing victory.

Look at this woman whose own doctor says she has, for the moment, "cheated death." They said the bad news was that she had six months to live, and there was no good news. Today, she's happier than she ever has been, ever. The angry person she was simply doesn't exist anymore. She has been physically transformed, down to the subatomic particles that make up every cell of her body. I admire her strength and her fearlessness. I have seen her heal on a physical, mental, and spiritual level. She is a living example of the possibilities inherent in all of us. What she has done, each and every one of us is capable of doing. It only takes commitment.

### THIRD CHAKRA EXERCISES
### SPINAL TWISTS FOR THE LIVER AND SPLEEN

1. Sit in an easy, cross-legged position on the floor.
2. Grasp your shoulders with your fingers in front, thumbs in back.
3. Inhale through your nose and twist to the left.
4. Exhale through your nose and twist to the right.
5. Inhale a silent "Sat" as you twist left, and exhale "Nam" as you twist right. Breathing should be long and deep. Eyes are closed.

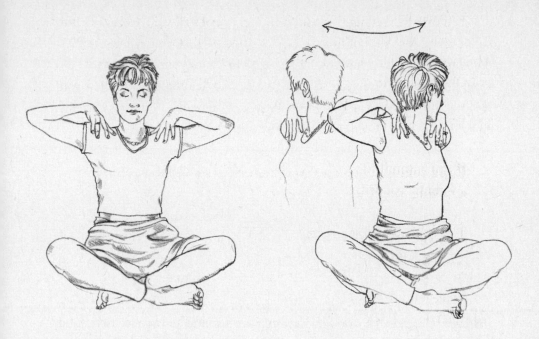

6. Continue twenty-six times at a smooth and moderate pace. Keep your arms parallel to the ground. End by inhaling facing forward. Relax.

## Exercise to Release Fear

1. Sit with the legs and arms extended straight in front of you. The arms are parallel to the ground, elbows straight.

2. Tightly fold the fingers onto the pads and point the thumbs straight up.

3. In this position, inhale through the nose, then exhale through the nose as you stretch forward, keeping the arms parallel to the ground.

4. Inhale back up into the beginning position with the back straight and perpendicular to the ground.

5. Use a heavy, powerful breath that gets heavier and heavier as you do this exercise.

6. Move rapidly, two breaths every five seconds. Remember to use the silent sounds of "Sat" on the inhale and "Nam" on the exhale.

7. Continue three to six minutes.

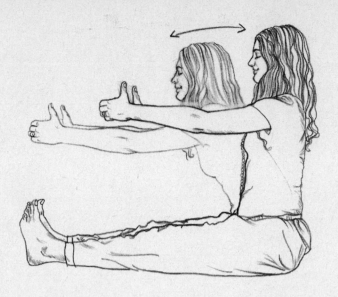

*Effects:* This exercise works on releasing the fear and tension we have stored up in our kidneys. It helps to give a gentle massage to the whole third chakra area, and all its related organs.

## ALTERNATE LEG LIFTS FOR STRENGTH AND DETERMINATION

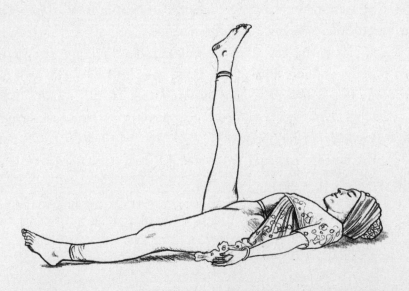

1. Lie flat on your back.

2. Inhale through the nose, lifting the right leg up to ninety degrees, with pointed toes. Keep the knee as straight as possible.

3. Exhale and lower it down.

4. Once the right leg touches the ground, repeat the sequence with the left leg.

5. Keep the breath powerful as you inhale "Sat" and exhale "Nam" ("I am Truth"). Remember, relax the shoulders.

6. Continue for three to eleven minutes.

If your lower back needs more support, place your hands, palms down, underneath your buttocks. You can also place a pillow under your neck for more support.

*Effects:* This exercise strengthens your abdominal muscles and your lower back, which in turn strengthens your will, determination, and commitment.

## STRESS-RELIEF MEDITATION

1. Sit in easy pose, in a comfortable, cross-legged position on the floor, and pull the spine straight.

2. Extend the right arm straight up in the air, hugging the right ear. The elbow is straight and the palm faces the left.

3. Extend the left arm up at a sixty-degree angle in front of you, the palm flat and face-down. Keep the elbow straight.

4. On both hands, put the thumbs onto the mound just below the little finger.

5. Inhale through the nose, "Sat." Exhale through the nose, "Nam."

6. Begin with three minutes. Gradually work up to eleven minutes. If you are not able to hold the arms up the entire time, bring them down, rest, and then go back up as many times as you need. You will heal no matter how many times your arms go up and down. As you go on, it becomes easier and you get stronger. This exercise is a challenge for everyone, including me!

7. Keep the eyes slightly open, looking down toward the upper lip.

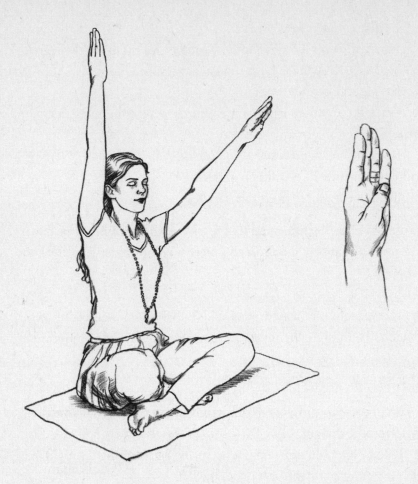

*Effects:* This meditation helps heal any weaknesses in the lower spine. It directly heals the kidneys and adrenal glands, helping to repair energy drained from long-term stress. It relaxes and rejuvenates the heart. There is no breath specified, but the breath will automatically become longer and deeper as you continue. Make sure you hold the arms perfectly still to receive the full benefits of this posture.

# 4

# The Fourth Chakra

COMPASSION

"The heart is the central place where the divinity of the Beloved exists. If you touch somebody's heart, it gets awakened."

—Yogi Bhajan

The fourth chakra is located in the physical body in the area of the heart and lungs, an area yogis often refer to as the heart center of the body, the heart chakra. It is one of the most powerful centers of the body, the home of compassion, which breeds kindness and goodwill to all. It is traditionally associated with the color green, and is fed by the earthly element, air. Your entire bloodstream pumps through this center, to nurture every organ of the body.

On the more etheric plane, the heavens and earth meet through this center. It is said that when we pray one prayer from the depths of our heart chakra, God has no choice but to listen and respond.

"Falling into prayer is exactly the same thing as falling in love. It is an infinite fall from which you never come out. These two experiences are the highest of all."

—Yogi Bhajan

Through this center of awareness, we move from "me" into the more universal realm of "we." Actually, the sound current often used to open and vibrate this chakra is "Hum," which literally means "we." It comes as no surprise that people traditionally associate the heart with the emotion of love. The overwhelming attraction of this chakra can be seen in our songs and sayings. Songs about the heart, the heart center, and love are very widespread. More has been written about love than almost any other human sentiment: "God is love," "Make love, not war," "Love is all you need," "Open up your heart, let the sunshine in," "I left my heart in San Francisco." We never sing songs about other organs, like the liver or the kidneys. You never hear a song like "I left my kidneys in San Francisco" or "Open up your liver and let the sunshine in." How do we begin to understand the talent that lies hidden in our fourth chakra and manifest it in our normal, everyday lives?

The heart radiates many emotions that are various expressions of love: warmth, compassion, passion, kindness, hatred. Every sentiment in the world emanates from the heart center. That is why it is the most powerful center and can be extremely dangerous if it is not guided by our intuition. *This is the center that gives life its richness, depth, and meaning.*

"We mess up our life mostly because of our heart.
This center controls passion.
Any time passion is not controlled by human intuition it will
bring destruction."

—Yogi Bhajan

Universal Love begins with compassion.

**"You shall understand another person's feeling accurately, intuitively, if you are compassionate."**

—Yogi Bhajan

Your heart center has a certain pulsation, a certain rhythm, which is so powerful that as much as you try to hide it, what you feel in your heart will show up on your face. If you learn how to speak and vibrate from this center, it is so magnetic that you can immediately convince another person of your opinions. This is because when you are truly vibrating from this center, you are not vibrating as "me" and "you"—you are vibrating as "we." The other person can feel his best interest, his needs, his very core being spoken to, even if only on an unconscious level. When the rhythm of your heart center is in harmony with another, you have not to speak one word, but that person will want to come and be with you.

Love has many facets. When the heart center is too active, a person may be overly sympathetic and forget to look after his own needs.

**"Your heart has not to open to others.
Your heart has to open to yourself."**

—Yogi Bhajan

When someone is imbalanced in this chakra, you may see him or her becoming overly attached to some object of affection. The emotion of fear is one darker side to the heart chakra that needs to be dealt with—fear of losing the object of your love, fear of caring for someone else and letting their needs override your own.

You might have heard the expression "Love your neighbor as yourself." Often people focus on only one side of this equation—the "love your neighbor" part—but they forget about the "love yourself" part. The saying doesn't read, "Love your neighbor more than yourself." It's "Love your neighbor AS yourself."

**"Self-rejection can bring you a lot of pain.
Learn to love yourself."**

—Yogi Bhajan

The wisdom in this simple equation is very profound, for it acknowledges that if you constantly put yourself down, refuse to take care of your physical body, ignore your legitimate needs, stuff away your feelings, in short . . .

**If you're not loving yourself, you won't be able to love others.**

With heart and lung disease and breast cancer alone, more people are suffering from diseases stemming from blockages or imbalances in this area of the body than in any other.

The purpose of this book is to give you simple, tangible tools to begin the healing process. Specifically with this energy center, the focus is to let go of the tension, let go of the fear, and let the heart open and bask in the warmth and feeling of well-being that comes when we experience real love.

During my thirty years of teaching the spiritual practice of Kundalini Yoga and Meditation, I have seen how people's emotional and spiritual blocks are made manifest in their bodies. I have felt the rock-hard, seized-up backs of heart patients. I often see students with unresolved issues develop diseases.

The idea that certain emotions can cause "dis-ease" in certain areas of our bodies is not a new one. An excess of a negative emotion prevailing in a certain chakra of our body is due to an imbalance in that chakra.

## COMPASSION

**"It is from a state of compassion that the healing activity of God within the being flows."**

**—Yogi Bhajan**

Love works best in our lives when expressed as compassion. "Love" can be a difficult word to understand, but "compassion" seems to express the more expanded, more universal side to love.

One of the things I love most about Kundalini Yoga and Meditation is that it's a practical way to love yourself. It doesn't have to be complicated, because loving yourself often begins with something as simple as allowing yourself one complete, deep breath.

It's just like those emergency instructions that flight attendants always give—to be sure that our own mask is firmly in place before assisting someone else with their oxygen mask. I remember as a young mother thinking that I couldn't do anything until I knew my baby was breathing; but, of course, that's not logical. I'm no good to my baby if I can't breathe and function. Apparently enough people make this logical error that the airlines feel they have to take the time to remind us of it every time we fly.

In the midst of panic and fear, you're not always able to see the importance of taking care of yourself. The truth is, if you're not good to yourself, you're no good to anyone else. Jesus certainly got it, and summed it up beautifully, "Love your neighbor AS yourself." Have compassion for your neighbor, have compassion for yourself.

How do we begin this process of having compassion for ourselves and others? The very beginning of making "love" an action word comes with the use of gratitude.

When I think of gratitude, I'm reminded of a story from my young adulthood. I was a hippie, a spiritual seeker living in Hawaii. This was during the sixties. My friends and I would often make flower leis and present them to visitors to the island as a welcoming gift. One day we gave flowers to a couple who seemed to radiate gratitude. They were sitting on a low stone wall, and the husband was very tender and attentive as he put the lei around his wife's neck. They thanked us profusely and seemed full of gratitude, for the beauty of Maui, for our kindness to them, and most of all for each other. I remember being so moved by their appreciation of each other.

All I remember to this day, more than thirty years later, was a radiant look on her face. What happened next surprised me. The husband got up to go. He picked his wife up in his arms. It was only then that I noticed that the woman was severely crippled, her legs were useless, and she had no arms, only useless little flipper-like appendages. I hadn't noticed this at all, even though it was obvious. I simply had not seen it. This couple's powerful aura of gratitude for what they did have blinded them and me to what was so obviously missing. Such is the power of gratitude.

God is love, and we are all created in the image of God, but that is an abstract idea. It's hard to think about God or love when I'm stuck in a long express checkout line at the market and the woman in front of me has more than twelve items. I could love her, but if I'm honest, I have to admit that mostly I am annoyed. She doesn't seem like God to me, and I'm not feeling too godly myself at that moment. [It's easy to see God when you're meditating on a mountain. It's a lot more challenging at the grocery store.] *hahaha!*
*TruthBomb!*

**"In love, your kindness and compassion have no limits."**

**—Yogi Bhajan**

Why am I annoyed with this woman in the grocery line? I am in a hurry and I don't feel as if I have enough time. I am coming from a place of want, from a poverty mentality. Since there isn't enough time, I feel that this woman is taking something away from me. In short, I am in fear. Love is the opposite of fear. Gratitude is the first step away from fear. It is almost impossible to be trapped in fear if you are really experiencing gratitude.

**"Recognize that the other person is you."**

**—Yogi Bhajan**

So how do I get to that place of gratitude, right there in the grocery line? As a yogi, I always begin on the physical level, because I know that's how I can learn to grow spiritually.

**I have often said to the students that what we do in class is the "practice" of yoga; life is the real yoga. In class we are practic-**

ing techniques, metaphorical life lessons on a physical level
that we can then apply to our larger lives in the world.

While I'm standing in the grocery line, I begin by examining how I
am standing, taking a moment to drop my shoulders. Chances are, they
are hovering around my ears. Then I close my eyes and use the yogic
technique of rolling my eyes up to the third eye point. In many cultures
the traditional posture of prayer involves putting the hands together and
pressing the thumbs to this place between the eyebrows. Try closing your
eyes and placing your hands in that traditional posture. When you have
done that, imagine that you are gazing up to that spot, even though your
eyes are closed. In doing this, you'll find that you feel an actual physical
sensation of relaxation.

The reasons for this are many. This area is the location of the pituitary gland, the gland that makes and regulates seratonin, the "feel-good
enzyme"; and focusing here stimulates seratonin production. Focusing
on the third eye point is one of the easiest and most effective ways to get
back on track, back in focus.

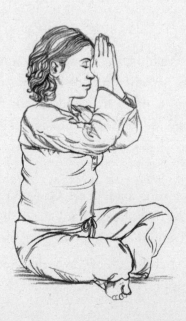

Having focused your eyes upward, already feeling calmer, inhale deeply through your nose, and as you inhale, think for a moment of something, anything for which you are grateful. It can be small or large; it can be the weather or your dog or the fact that you have a warm, safe place to sleep and good food to eat. Anything at all. Hold the breath and that thought for a few seconds. As you exhale slowly, again through your nose, consciously breathe away one specific thing that you are afraid of, letting it go out on your exhale. In that exhale, for those few moments, agree to give that fear over to God. You don't have to give it away forever. If you want to worry about it some more, you can have it back, but for those few seconds, trust God to take care of your mortgage, job, family, and health.

## THE GRATITUDE EXERCISE

1. Inhale through the nose.
2. Exhale completely through the mouth.
3. Inhale deeply and smoothly through the mouth.
4. Exhale completely through the nose.
5. Continue, inhaling the mantra "Sat" and exhaling the mantra "Nam."

*Effects:* This simple breath meditation will help you to overcome any animosity, and turn these emotions into compassion instead. Once finished, silently say "thank you" to the woman who has too many items in her basket, for almost miraculously you are grateful for her giving you the opportunity to meditate. Then when she goes to pay by check, you won't even react!

**"If somebody is terribly bad, thank God that it is not you. And if somebody is terribly good, thank God that you have seen something good, and that it could be you, too."**

**—Yogi Bhajan**

## FEAR AND ATTACHMENT

One shadow emotion of the heart center is that of fear and attachment.

Fear is very visibly present in our Western society. Fear marks the body in the area of the heart and chest. The heart chakra crisis in our society is why we are suffering from an epidemic of the "disease of fear." When you consider heart disease, lung disease, and breast cancer, fear is the number one premature killer.

> **"There are two forces which work in life — love and fear.**
> **Love and fear are two sides of the same coin.**
> **Therefore if you are afraid, remember, it's a moving force to be**
> **dealt with."**
>
> **—Yogi Bhajan**

Doing physical and spiritual work to get from a place of fear into a place of gratitude will change your life and your health for the better. I've seen it time and time again.

Many people's greatest fear is the fear of death and dying, confronting the unknown, what we will go through in the dying process and when it will occur. It's also our most realistic fear, because it's an experience that everyone will eventually have to face and go through. Specifically, we fear the pain of dying and the uncertainty of when death will happen to us. On a logical level, it's easy to accept that it's foolish to fear the one thing that is guaranteed to happen, but accepting that emotionally is perhaps the greatest challenge of being human. As yogis, we say you will die, but you never have to grow old. We come to go.

> **"Death is just shedding your body. It is like taking off your**
> **shirt and throwing it away.**
> **So why are we so afraid?**
> **At the time of death, the entire life you have lived is**

panoramically shown to you, and you are made the judge.
If you can *forgive* yourself at that time, you are liberated."
—Yogi Bhajan

In my many years of working with cardiac patients, I have seen the effect that fear has on our physical body.

"Death is not unimportant or important—but FEAR is very
important.
Any moment of life is a dead moment when you are not at
your highest frequency.
To die is an art.
Great are those who have learned to die with smiles on their
faces."
—Yogi Bhajan

I have taught yoga workshops for cardiac surgery patients from Cedar Sinai Hospital in Los Angeles. Almost without exception, there was a marked tightness in the upper backs of these patients, a clenching of the muscles. This is the body's desperate and misguided attempt to shield the heart.

When these patients begin doing yoga, making even the smallest effort to open this area physically, it becomes easier for them to open themselves emotionally and spiritually to their recovery. Patients began experiencing gratitude, making changes in their work lives, cutting back, realizing what really mattered to them. I have often felt that a heart attack can be a beautiful wake-up call from your heart. Your heart is saying, "Honor me. Love me. I am yours."

A student once told me a wonderful story that expresses how confronting fear, accepting it, feeling it, and moving through it can change your life. The story takes place during a devastating hurricane on Cape Cod in the 1950s. A woman who lived alone in a house on a bay had decided to ride out the hurricane, even though everyone had been told to evacuate. She was too afraid of leaving, so much did her possessions, her home, mean to her. Unfortunately, the storm was worse than anyone could imagine. By the time she realized that she should get out, all the roads were flooded.

The woman got word by radio that a tidal surge was coming. She knew that the wave was big enough to engulf her house. Her first impulse was to lock up the house tightly and hope for the best, but logically she knew that this enormous wall of water would break the windows. The water would pour in, and everything she owned would be ruined. Her home would be destroyed by the force of the water, and she would surely be killed.

Then she had a flash of inspiration. What if, instead of trying to fight this enormous force, she accepted it, faced directly the thing she feared most? And that is exactly what she did. She opened every door and window in her house, and she climbed up on her roof. When the wave came, she actually dived with it, allowing it to carry her to eventual safety.

Amazingly, her house was also saved, because the house did not offer resistance. The water flowed through, destroying her possessions but allowing the house to stand. All the other houses on the point were destroyed, and many people were killed, but she survived. She let go of her attachment, her denial, accepted what was really happening, survived, and thrived. She lived to be a very elderly lady, happy in that house for many years.

This story is such a wonderful metaphor for accepting that life is scary, and there are things beyond our control. What this woman literally did was to take the proverbial "leap of faith."

Fortunately, most life situations are not this dramatic. Most of the time, the fear we face is not catastrophic, it's claustrophobic. Everyday fears that usually come in the form of worry—low-grade, never-ending series of niggling, nagging possibilities we play out in our minds of the things that could go wrong. The "what ifs" that awaken you at three A.M. and keep you from going back to sleep.

It's important to remember that worrying is an activity; it is a choice.

People often say, "I am worried," as though it is something that is being done to them, something over which they have no control—but that's not accurate. It's more accurate to say, "I am worrying," because it is something I do by choice.

> **"What gives you strength? Your thoughts.**
> **What weakens you? Your thoughts.**
> **What destroys you? Your thoughts.**
> **In reality, thoughts are given to expand you, so you'll realize,**
> **'I am All.'"**
>
> **—Yogi Bhajan**

Until we have experienced worry as a choice, these are just words and the truth of someone else. Even if you accept that, you may be saying, "Fine, great, but how do I make the choice to stop worrying? It seems to happen before I know it, and I don't know how to stop." It's true that in every blink of the eye a thousand thoughts pass through your mind, but to which do you gravitate most? Usually to the negative ones, because the pull to the negative is many times stronger than to the positive.

> **"Your brain will release thoughts,**
> **one thousand per wink of the eye.**
> **So you have no thinking power.**
> **You only have a PURSUING power.**
> **It is up to you which thoughts you will pursue."**
>
> **—Yogi Bhajan**

Your mind is like a dog. It can be trained, and it can be trained best by using love, praise, and affection.

Attitude is important. The "attitude of gratitude" looks to how we can change a pattern in the body first, and then use that physical adjustment to help alter our mental, emotional, and spiritual reaction.

**Happiness is your birthright.**

Happiness can become your norm rather than the exception. Even the most spiritual people who have ever lived—Jesus, Buddha, Mohammed, Yogi Bhajan, all the saints and sages and teachers—regardless of their level of enlightenment, experienced pain, sorrow, and grief.

**Pain is part of life. We are not human beings having a spiritual experience; we are spiritual beings having a human experience.**

Through your physical body you have the human experience. People who have had a near-death experience describe the feeling of leaving their bodies as a tremendous freedom, a feeling of pure joy. Clearly, when we are pure spirit, joy is our natural state. You don't own your body, you lease it, and at the end of the lease you turn it in. So, it follows, why do we come into our bodies?

We have all heard the expression "My body is a temple." We come into our bodies so we can experience more fully love for the Creator. Your body is the temple in which you learn to love God. Yoga, yogic healing, and meditation are tools to help you.

**Yoga is not a religion; it is a practice. Literally the word "yoga" means "a yoke that brings union." It means bringing the finite (your body) into the Infinite (your consciousness).**

Yoga is a discipline that can become an extension of your chosen faith or belief system. I am an American Sikh. That is my faith. Yoga is a tool that helps me to redefine my relationship with the Creator.

**"There's a difference between religion and yoga.
Religion gives you a hope: 'Lean on God and keep moving.'
Yoga says, 'God is in you; lean on your Self and move on.'
That's the difference between the two philosophies."**
**—Yogi Bhajan**

One of the things I love about yoga as a spiritual tool is its practicality and its simplicity. I have students of almost every faith—Christian, Muslim,

Hindu, Jewish, Sikh, Bahai, Shinto, Buddhist—and those of no set faith. All of them use their yogic practice as a way of enhancing their chosen path.

There are a million wonderful books that can inspire you with ways to live a more spiritual life. And there is truth in all of them, but how do we do it? Kundalini Yoga and Meditation offer more than inspiration. Worrying is a low-grade form of fear. Fear keeps us from loving, while gratitude brings us into love. So how do we make gratitude the attitude? If you are worrying, take a moment and become aware of your tongue.

When you are worrying, the tongue is the first muscle in your body that will tense up. The minute it does, it throws off your breathing and the heart center.

Wherever you are, close your eyes, drop your jaw, and let your tongue hang out. Inhale through your nose, exhale through your mouth, letting the tongue totally go limp. When I have my hands on a student's shoulders who is doing this, it's amazing what happens. Immediately their shoulders drop, the back of the heart center opens, the rib cage relaxes, thus increasing the space for the lungs to expand. The pulse slows, the blood pressure often drops. It's astonishing. It's almost as though your tongue is an amazing on-off switch.

Even better than letting your tongue hang out is to accompany it with a sound. As you exhale, softly make the sound "Ahhh." If you are somewhere where people won't think you're crazy, you can make it a very loud "Ahhh!" And really, who cares if people think you're crazy? I love doing this exercise, because I think of being in gratitude as being in a state of awe, and making the sound of "Ahhh!" physically reminds me of that idea.

Also, as your tongue becomes more relaxed, you'll find you won't say words you want to take back. You'll find your swearing will lessen and your food choices will be more fresh and alive. Try this for a few minutes. Inhale through your nose, let your tongue hang out, and as you exhale, make the sound "Ahhh."

When I teach, I talk the students through an exercise, so let's try it here.

## THE ANTI-WORRY EXERCISE

1.   Sit in a comfortable cross-legged position (easy pose), with a straight spine.

2.   Place the palms flat together with the fingers extended.

3.   With the elbows straight, extend the arms sixty degrees up in the air and as far to the left as possible. The upper right arm will extend right below your chin.

4.   Keep the eyes closed.

5.   The fingertips of the right hand cover the mounds at the base of the fingers of the left hand. Be sure to keep the elbows stretched out and up and locked throughout the meditation.

6.   Inhale powerfully and deeply through the nose; and exhale powerfully through the mouth, pressing the navel deeply in toward the spine. Concentrate on your breath.

7.   Hold the position for three, seven, or eleven minutes.

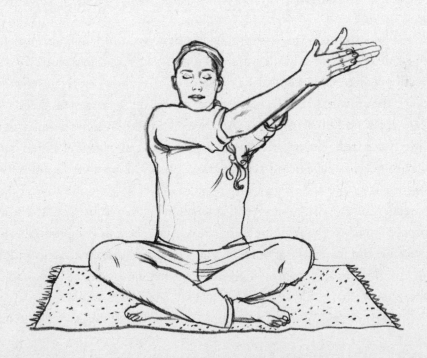

8. At the end of the meditation, inhale very deeply, then exhale very powerfully, holding the breath out for ten to fifteen seconds. Inhale and relax.

*Effects:* This meditation is good for anyone who worries. It releases tension and helps alleviate depression. The shoulders and elbows may ache as the body corrects itself, but keep the elbows locked, regardless! It is good for people who have any kind of heart problem.

How important is this thing you are worried about? How important is it, viewed in the scope of your whole human experience?

There is no right answer to this question. What you're worried about may be the most crucial thing that's ever happened to you. Most of the time it's not as important as it seems, and even if it is the most important thing that is happening to you in your whole life, worrying will never bring the outcome for which you're longing.

Do you think that God has made a mistake in putting this challenge in your life?

If the answer to this question is no, then give this challenge over to the care of God to solve in ways you might never, ever conceive. God's plans are often far better than our own.

If the answer is "Yes, God has in fact made a mistake, and God doesn't care about me," that's fine, too. We have all felt this at some point in our lives. Jesus said, "Father, why has Thou forsaken me?" Everyone feels that way sometimes. The act of acknowledging that feeling, that doubt, is the beginning of the path from worry to gratitude. If we take the case of the teacher Jesus, we can remember that by realizing his doubt, he was able to accept those who nailed him to the cross. After accepting, he moved into gratitude and release. "It is finished, into Thy hands I commend my spirit."

Many times in counseling families who have a loved one going through an illness, I have heard doctors say, "We've done all we can; now we leave the rest to God." I laugh. Where did they think God was all along?

Keep up the wonderful breath pattern, inhale deeply, tongue out, exhale, "Ahhh." When I think about the feeling that God has forgotten me, I am reminded of a story a student told me about her dog. She had a beautiful Doberman who was an angel in her life. She was a person who tended to be very cynical, and she loved how her dog seemed to be a devout optimist. To that dog, anything could be a sign that a walk was about to take place. A walk was pure heaven on earth to that sweet Dobie. If the student changed her clothes or hung up the phone or opened the front door, any of those things could mean that a walk was about to happen, and her dog always believed in the possibility of that happy outcome. She was God to that dog. As far as the dog was concerned, God was good, God would always provide.

The dog became ill. She developed a horrible infection in her hind leg and had to be kept as immobile as possible to try to save her leg. If the infection could not be healed, the leg would have to be amputated. The dog wasn't allowed to go on walks for five months, and previously she had gone for a walk almost every day. For a while the dog kept hoping that the walk would come, but it never did. The dog seemed to become depressed, began ripping up the sofa, eating shoes. The dog felt that "God," in the form of her mistress, had forsaken her.

My student had no way to communicate the bigger picture to the dog. She was actually loving her pet and caring for her so that she would one day be able to run and jump and play.

When I think back on the times in my life when it seemed that God had forsaken me, I now realize that I, just like the dog, had no way of being able to see the bigger picture. When I think God has forgotten me, God may actually be protecting or teaching me.

Eventually the dog healed. Today she has all four legs and runs and jumps and plays.

Back to our tongue exercise. Continue inhaling through the nose and exhaling through the mouth, relaxing the tongue more with every breath, making the sound of "Ahhh." And now answer these questions: What does the worry get me? How important is it?

**Is this problem too big for God? God never gives us more than we can handle.**

Do this exercise all the time. Sometimes in a stressful situation, excuse yourself, go to the public bathroom in a stall, close your eyes, relax your tongue. Ask these questions of yourself and finish by taking a deep breath and saying out loud, "Thank you, God." Exhale completely that one breath, and then go on with your day. It's a practical tool, returning you back to your center.

Guess what you just did? A Kundalini Yoga exercise and meditation for the heart chakra—a meditation to increase your experience of opening the gratitude in your heart.

It's a challenge to feel gratitude when you are tired and resentful. Try playing a little game based on one we'd play as kids. When we used to drive in the car, we'd play, "A—my name is Alice." You remember that game: You have to go through the whole alphabet saying, "A—my name is Alice, my husband's name is Arthur. We live in Alaska. We sell artichokes." The grown-up version of this game is to go through the alphabet and for every letter, name something you are grateful for, whether it's huge or trivial. Due to the nature of the game, I probably expressed more gratitude for zebras and xylophones than anything else on earth, but you know what? I AM grateful for xylophones, and who wouldn't be grateful for the beautiful zebra?

Whenever I play this little game, I unfailingly feel better than when I started. Being grateful for twenty-six things can definitely free you from your fears.

## FOURTH CHAKRA EXERCISES
## EXERCISE TO OPEN YOUR HEART

1.    Begin by stretching your arms out in front of you with your palms pressed firmly together, elbows straight, arms parallel to the floor.

2.    As you inhale deeply through your nose, open your arms out wide

in a large, expansive gesture. Feel the area of your heart center open and expand as your lungs fill with air. Your arms keep opening and stretching, eventually stretching back as far as they can go. Really feel the stretch as though your arms were giant wings you are stretching in the bright morning sun. Feel the stretch across your chest, under the arms, under your ribs, down the arms, and out through the fingertips. Keep the arms parallel to the ground the entire time.

3.   When your arms are stretched open as wide as they can go, feel your shoulder blades almost touching each other. Begin exhaling power-fully through your nose, and bring your arms back to the original position, ending with your palms pressed together once again.

4.   Do the movement as pictured twenty-six times, with your eyes closed and rolled up to your third eye point the entire time. Remember to inhale deeply and exhale powerfully, silently reciting "Sat" on the inhale and "Nam" on the exhale. Sat Nam means "I am Truth" or "Truth is my True Identity." Move at a moderate pace.

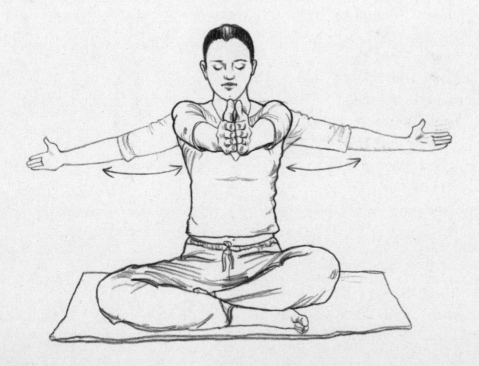

*Effects:* This Kundalini Yoga exercise is a very simple movement, but it has an amazing effect in opening the heart center.

### MEDITATION FOR THE HEART CENTER

1.  Sit in easy pose, with the legs crossed, spine straight.
2.  Extend your arms straight out to the sides, parallel to the ground. Bend the elbows so the forearms form a ninety-degree angle straight up. The palms are flat and facing forward.
3.  Close your eyes, rolling them up to the third eye point. Inhale deeply through your nose, and as you exhale make the sound "Hummmmm." Really allow this very healing sound current to resonate through your face, beginning with your lips, which should be pressed together gently like two petals.

*Effects:* Chanting "Humm" is what we refer to in yoga as a mantra. It is a healing sound we use in meditation. It is through this sound current, which

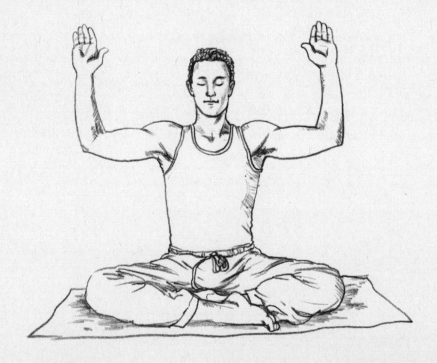

means "we," that we move from individual consciousness into divine love, connecting to the Infinite through our heart center.

Start out doing this meditation for three minutes, then build it up to seven, eleven, or even thirty-one minutes. I do promise you that even after three minutes, this amazing resonance of sound within your body will begin to work its healing magic. It's such a beautiful way to begin the process of taking care of yourself.

# 5
# The Fifth Chakra

TRUTH

"Whatever the strength of your tongue, that is your universe."

—Yogi Bhajan

The fifth human talent, the talent of truth, is contained in your throat chakra. This area includes the neck, the shoulders, the mouth, the nose, and the ears—the gateway between the head and the heart. It is here we learn what is our own authentic voice—what we are meant to "say to the world" during our time here on earth.

When I was in my early twenties, I worked in the theater as an actress, and I remember a director telling me, "Just be yourself," as if that were the easiest thing in the world to do! I had no idea how to do that, and it terrified me. Now I think that to "just be yourself" may be the *healthiest* thing in the world to do—but what does it mean?

**The practice of Kundalini Yoga and Meditation provides tools that let our authentic voices emerge from whatever false identities we may have taken on, consciously or unconsciously.**

In my years of teaching and listening to students, I have learned to hear when people are stuck in unhealthy patterns. I can literally hear it in the voice. Perhaps one of the easiest examples of this is something most people find annoying, the habit of "baby talk" to another adult, usually a lover. The relationship is being forged to replace affection that wasn't received in childhood. This expresses itself when the lovers speak as babies to each other. It may indeed heal an old wound, but it doesn't ring true to the ear because the voices heard are not in the present.

**One of the greatest ways to tap into the truth of who you really are is to begin working with and loving your own human voice.**

When I teach "Mommy and Me Yoga" I look out over a sun-filled studio of twenty or thirty mothers and their babies. Some of the babies nap, some howl, some gurgle and coo, some are nursing. The sights and sounds of that class always fill me with a great sense of contentment, especially since I've usually known most of those babies since they were in the womb, and they always seem to recognize my voice. I am constantly amazed at the symphony of baby sounds. Babies are in love with the sound of their own voice, and happy to use their full and glorious range.

I have a student who is a singing teacher who has told me that the most perfectly produced vocal sound is the wail of an infant. Even highly trained opera singers cannot support a tone for the length (or at the decibel level) of a tiny baby. Anyone who has ever been awakened for a four A.M. feeding would certainly have to agree with her. Of course, babies don't disguise their feelings; they "speak up for themselves" with complete honesty. Slowly, as we get older, we lose that ability. So many of us speak in an adult monotone that sounds very much like the "wah wah wah wah" of the adults in the *Peanuts* animated series. It's just what happens to us. It is all patterning from when we were in our mother's womb, and during the first three years of our lives.

I'm not suggesting that we all go back to wailing our heads off. In order to begin to regain your authentic voice on an everyday basis, I do know that nothing can help release stress and tension better than a little yogic vocalizing.

**"This world is ruled by the word, and whosoever's word is shallow, that person is shallow."**

**—Yogi Bhajan**

EXERCISE
DOG BREATH
In Kundalini Yoga, there is a supremely healing breath pattern called "Dog Breath."

1. Sit with your mouth open, extend your tongue out as far as it will go, and pant rapidly like a dog. Pant fast and deeply, putting the power of

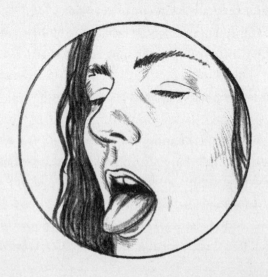

the diaphragm and navel into it. As the breath comes in, the navel moves out. As the breath goes out, the navel moves in.

2.   Pump your belly. After a minute and a half, allow the sound of your panting to move back down into your throat, becoming more guttural.

3.   Do this for three minutes.

*Effects:* This breath pattern will help clear your body and throat chakra of toxins. It helps to super-oxygenate your blood if you are feeling run-down. It is said to help get rid of viral diseases, as well as open up areas of your brain to increase intuition. It will help you to clear out old lies and fears and leave you with speaking your truth.

**"When you speak, it should be as if Infinity is speaking."**
—Yogi Bhajan

## SINGING

The reason singing has such a powerful pull on our inner selves is because when we sing even the simplest song, we are more in touch with our soul. All singers are "soul singers." When you hold a new baby in your arms, humming and cooing and singing to it are the most natural things in the world to do. We need to keep singing those little lullabies and tunes every day, especially to ourselves. My teacher Yogi Bhajan has said many times that a family that sings together, and thus a nation that sings together, will bring peace on earth.

A dear friend of mine who is originally from Greece told me that in her country, people often sing aloud in public, in the street, or in a restaurant. When they break into song, others just join in with them. That sounds so wonderful to me, like those great old movie musicals I loved as a kid. My friend now lives in South Africa, and says you hear people singing in public there all the time, too. I know that people in America are usually too embarrassed to sing in the streets. It's great that we at least allow ourselves to sing in the car. I just love it when I'm stopped at a light and in my rearview mirror I see someone singing. It just makes my day to see the joy on his face. The act of singing truly heals us all.

I started to understand the power of singing to ourselves as a way of healing when I was looking through old family snapshots one day. The people in the pictures seemed visibly happier, more radiant, when they were photographed singing "Happy Birthday." The same people would look completely different in a picture that might have been snapped just a few moments before they started singing. Once they start singing, the people seemed more filled with light. And no, it isn't just the effect of the candles on the cake.

The reason for this remarkable transformation was the very act of singing itself. When we are doing something as simple as singing "Happy Birthday," it is actually a powerful tool that helps to remove our everyday self-imposed limitations. It returns us to our days in infancy when we made sounds just for the sheer joy of it. Lifting voices in song has been a way of reaching the God within us for as long as humans have been on the earth, and that is why singing is part of Kundalini Yoga.

**The human voice is designed to sing, and our soul is a song in our hearts that must be heard.**

Even if you cannot carry a tune, start singing. Once the throat chakra opens and connects with the heart, you will be able to sing in tune, because the broken bridge between the two will be healed. Your voice will begin to sing the song of your soul.

We always sing a simple little song at the end of every Kundalini Yoga class, all over the world. It has been translated in many languages. There are other meditations for which we use the words of a simple children's song, like "Row, row, row your boat, gently down the stream. Merrily, merrily, merrily, merrily, life is but a dream." These are very truthful words; within them lies a message as old as human existence.

Many students will roll their eyes at first, obviously wondering how they ended up rolling around on the floor singing songs they learned on the playground. I see this especially during pregnancy workshops when the husbands come for the first time to do yoga with their pregnant wives, who are already used to the unusual. But very quickly they lose themselves in the fun of a sing-along, regardless of how difficult the posture. Shoulders and necks relax, eyes brighten, mouths begin to smile. I always see the "Happy Birthday Effect" take place.

> **"Words are not a small thing. Words are the real power.**
> **The whole universe is a magnetic field.**
> **If we create positive words, we feel love.**
> **If we create negative words, we feel hatred."**
>
> **—Yogi Bhajan**

My sister teaches in the Waldorf School system, in which children sing little songs guiding them through their daily tasks. "The Hand Washing Song," "The Getting Dressed Song"—all these little tunes have a marvelous, relaxing, positive effect on the kids. Using songs in your life will have the same effect on you. Music conductors are some of the longest-living people on earth—standing right in the middle of this glorious sound current.

> **"Communication is a gift to know, to understand and a gift to**
> **realize.**
> **Let your words be straight, simple, and said with a smile."**
>
> **—Yogi Bhajan**

Now, you may be thinking, "Why on earth do I need this woman to tell me to breathe deeply, lower my shoulders, sing a silly song?" It's a good question. The practice of yoga and meditation is often simple, which people misinterpret as being simple-minded. Our modern world is so complex, it often gives us an unnatural craving for complex solutions. But once we get past our ego's need for complex solutions, we accept that our problems are no more complicated than the problems of any other person. All our life problems are not complex; some are really incredibly simple. Once we have accepted that possibility, we realize that simple tools often work. Some of these tools are the practices of prayer, yoga, meditation, going to church or synagogue, as well as therapy and other support groups. Or your tools can be something else altogether, like cooking dinner for your family and friends, taking a walk, or buying a gift for a friend. Every day, begin simply.

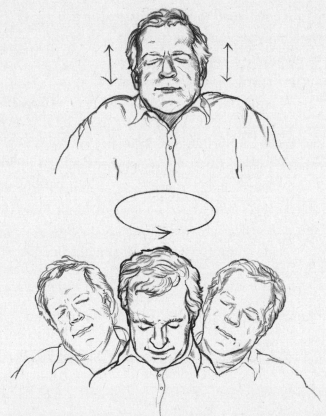

## MEDITATION ON THE INFINITE SOUND CURRENT OF "ONG"

1. Breathe in and out deeply through your nose a few times.
2. Scrunch your shoulders up tightly to your ears, and then relax and lower your shoulders. Do this five times.

3. Then close your eyes and roll your head around—first to the right, and then to the left, inhaling and exhaling through the nose deeply.

4. Bring your head straight up, and roll the eyes up to the third eye point. Let your hands relax in your lap.

5. Then bring the head straight up and chant, "Ong." Curl the tongue and press the back of the tongue against the back of the throat firmly.

6. Do this for three to seven minutes.

*Effects:* It will sound as if you are singing through your nose, "Onnnnng." You will begin to feel a slight buzz in the area where the root of your nose and the back of the throat meet. "Ong" means "Infinity" in its most creative form, and chanting this sound is very relaxing and uplifting.

A survey was published recently that asked the following question: "If you could ask God just one question and get a definitive answer, what question would you ask?" Much to my surprise, no one asked if Elvis was really dead. Some people wanted to know if there was life after death, but by far the question most asked was "What is the purpose of my life? What is God's plan for me?"

Clearly, people feel that God does have a plan for their lives, and they would love to know more about what that plan is. The beginning of that answer comes in sitting still. If you sit still, God will come to you. In fact, everything will.

There's an old folk tale that I love; I remember it being read to me as a child. I have no idea from where it came. I just remember that it was in an old picture book, and that the illustrations looked dark and Germanic, so I always see this story taking place in a deep Bavarian forest.

The story goes like this: A husband and wife were very unhappy and fought bitterly. They were poor, and they struggled and constantly blamed each other for their problems. They never believed that anything would ever get better. Then one day a sparkling magic wizard appeared to them and granted them three wishes. The husband and the wife pooh-poohed the idea. Life was hard and bitter, and there was no such thing as wishes and magic, so why even bother? But the wizard insisted they try it, just to see if they had the power to wish for whatever they wanted.

Finally the wife said, "Fine, I wish that my husband would have a giant sausage for a nose," and *poof*, so he did.

Rather than be amazed that they did in fact have the power to transform their miserable lives, the husband became furious with his wife and shouted, "Fine! I wish that my wife would have an even bigger sausage for a nose!" and *poof*, so she did.

Now they only had one wish left, and they had to use that wish to remove their big sausage noses.

By our words we do make things so. With real commitment that the power of how we speak affects our body, our mind, and our spirit, then and only then will we begin to transform our lives through the power of the word. The soul's voice rings clear like a bell.

**"There is a saying that the cut from a sword can be stitched and healed, but the cut of a tongue can never be."**

—Yogi Bhajan

I had a student who tried an experiment. She was the sort of person who constantly put herself down and didn't even realize it. Every time she said something like "I'm so stupid," she forced herself reflexively to say the exact opposite: "I'm smart." She said she felt silly doing it, but she did it. She cured herself of the habit of saying negative things about herself.

**"When a negative thought hits you, hit it with a positive thought—you will come out the best."**

—Yogi Bhajan

I have a dear doctor friend. Whenever I asked him how it was going, he would almost always say, "Gurmukh, it's really hard." One day in a soft moment, I approached him with the idea of eliminating that expression from his vocabulary for forty days, just to see what would happen in his life. It was an incredible discipline for him to let go of these words, but he did it, and his life and practice both improved! He was amazed, and has not used these words since.

**You are what you say.**

Here's another experiment you can try. Say, "I want." Listen to the sound of your voice saying those words. You can even tape-record it if you like. And then try saying, "I am." You probably will sound more relaxed when you say, "I am." The words we say do matter, and they resonate powerfully within our bodies. Cruel words spoken or heard actually do cellular damage to our living tissues. It's a damage that can be repaired, but it takes conscious effort. When you say, "I am," you empower yourself with self-acceptance and love. When you say, "I want," you are saying, "I am not enough the way I am. Until this want is met, I cannot love myself and my life totally."

**The words we say do matter, and they resonate powerfully within our bodies.**

To open your throat chakra and develop your ability to speak the truth, I recommend the use of chanting, which is different from singing. Chanting is simply the act of repeating a series of sounds over and over that make us feel better and more relaxed. It is particularly healing for our throat chakra and for the entire body. The sounds send messages to our brains that reinforce the positive and heal old wounds within our cellular coding.

EXERCISE
CHANTING "SAT NAM" TO OPEN THE
THROAT CHAKRA

1.  Sit quietly.
2.  Close your eyes and focus on the third eye point.
3.  Inhale deeply. On the exhale, begin singing out the sounds "Sat

Nam." When chanting "Sat Nam," chant the "Sat" really long and the "Nam" very short, dropping the tone a half note.

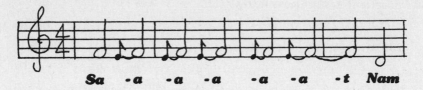

*Effects:* Chanting three to five minutes a day, "Sat Nam" ("I am Truth") is just one of the many tools that can help us open our throat chakra and connect with the universal Truth. This leads to huge life changes in beginning to understand who we are and what we are to do with our precious time on the planet.

When a healing practice can be found to have existed for thousands of years in various cultures, it must have some validity. Chanting exists in cultures throughout the world. It is part of the Hindu, Catholic, Sufi, Native American, Aboriginal, Sikh, Buddhist, and every other tradition.

**Chanting for even just three or five minutes a day is one of the many tools that can help us open up our throat chakra and connect with our human talent of truth.**

It's wonderful that so many people in the Western medical community are beginning to acknowledge the potential in tools like chanting for healing disease. For example, people like Mitchell Gaynor, M.D., who is the director of oncology and integrative medicine at the Strang Cancer Prevention Center in New York City, has been working with chanting and meditation for his cancer patients with astounding results.

In his book *Sounds of Healing: A Physician Reveals the Therapeutic Power of Sound, Voice and Music,* he discusses the healing power of sound. He claims that since the body is seventy percent water, and since sound is conducted easily through water, that is how sound heals on a cellular level. He even cites a recent study in which critical-care heart patients were monitored to reveal that thirty minutes of music therapy had the same physical effect of calming stress as did a ten-milligram dose of Valium.

These kinds of studies only reconfirm what I know to be true from almost thirty years of working with people. Sound current, meditation, yoga, breath patterns—these various techniques *do* work in reducing tension, strengthening the body, and comforting the soul. When people begin to use them on even the smallest level, their lives change. I see it every day. In fact, it has been the joy of my life to be a part of spreading the word, showing students how to restore that natural balance of serenity that is within every one of us.

Disciplining yourself to doing something that will change your brain patterning may not prove to be an easy or pain-free process. There's always going to be a part of your subconscious that will fight the healing, fight letting go of the old. But being stuck in negative patterns is more painful. Growth is never pain-free.

**I believe that anyone who promises you change that is pain-free is trying to sell you a lie.**

I have seen people begin to discover their truth, to find out what it is they really want to do with their lives, only to discover that their spouses, friends, and family are afraid of the changes. That is a challenge. Most of us are patterned to think of change as loss.

**Although it cannot be denied, sometimes there is loss with change; clinging to something familiar that is not healthy for you will never bring happiness.**

The people who really love you will eventually realize that you need to be your most authentic self. Try to remember that anyone who doesn't love you when you are being the best person you know how to be, might be somebody who is really not your friend.

Losing what is familiar, no matter how detrimental it may have been for us, is more than some people can bear. Finding yourself shouldn't mean losing the people in your life.

Another phenomenon occurs when a person begins a path of yoga and self-improvement work. Part of growth requires looking at yourself, viewing your own shortcomings, and taking responsibility to change them or not. At times our unconscious will begins to balk, if the change is happening too fast or becomes too intense. Sometimes at this point a person will look for the source of his discomfort in someone or something outside of himself, rather than deal with his own internal conflicts. Sometimes people, often unconsciously, decide that it is easier and more comfortable to blame someone else than to make real changes in their own character. This is the "What's wrong with me is actually you" syndrome.

We live in a culture of blame. In our justice system, we see murderers arguing that sugar or alcohol, or even premenstrual syndrome, made them commit their crimes. The effect of all this blaming is that it turns everyone into a victim. No one can address his or her problems if they believe they are someone else's fault. If you are unhappy in any area of your life, you are the one who needs to change. In order to break the cycle of blame, we need to turn the focus back onto ourselves.

**Learn to give up blame so that you can find your own truth and live it.**

A student told me a story the other day that perfectly illustrated how not speaking our truth harms us. She was working in a restaurant as a cook. She had been very unhappy in the job, although she liked the work. The source of her unhappiness, she thought, was the owner, who was very sarcastic and loved to humiliate her employees. When my student burned some fish she was cooking, her boss deluged her with her usual torrent of sarcasm. The student offered to pay for the damaged food and the boss took her up on it, further humiliating her by forcing her to get the money out of her wallet. She decided to quit. She told her decision to someone else in the kitchen, avoiding her boss.

When she got home that very evening, she began to develop a fearsome sore throat, the kind that prevents you from swallowing. Since she had been a yoga student for a while, she began thinking about her throat chakra, and not speaking her truth. She realized that by avoiding her boss and not speaking her truth, she was getting a sore throat. This had been a pattern of hers.

The next day, she went back to the restaurant and spoke to her boss personally. The discussion was not confrontative. The student just told her boss the reason she was quitting was she couldn't take being humiliated any more. The boss began to cry and asked the student if she thought this was why she had such a terrible turnover of employees. The student replied that yes, everyone who had quit left because of the boss's vicious sarcasm. My student didn't end up going back to the job, since she had already accepted another. But the moment she left the restaurant, after hugs and tears from her boss, her sore throat was completely gone. By speaking truth, she had healed herself and helped another human being.

**We are powerless over every other person on the planet, and we only have power over our own lives. No matter how problematic the people in your life are, you are always the solution.**

You can't change anyone else, and even if you miraculously could, you would still be the main challenge in your own life. Your Monkey Mind is the challenge, but you, in partnership with God, are also the solution to any troubles you may have. You are your own best healer. As in the case of the student and her boss, in the end she saw it wasn't the boss who was her problem. This student's fear was her own worst problem. She had been untruthful to herself by remaining in a work environment that was harmful to her. Until she was honest about why she had to go, she was not going to be fully healed.

There is another student who is going through what I see as a throat chakra crisis as this book is being written. She is in a fifteen-year marriage. Her husband is a very successful executive who has recently gotten sober. In this relationship, which in many ways is very loving, there has also been a lot of "asleepness" on both of their parts. Both partners are beginning to tell the truth.

Although it is painful, these two people are beginning to heal themselves and their marriage. In addition to using the tools of the twelve-step programs, Alcoholics Anonymous and Al-Anon, as well as couples counseling, this student has been practicing yoga and meditation and finds that it enhances everything else she is doing at this crisis point. She says learning to speak her truth by acknowledging the harmful patterns that exist in this relationship both in Al-Anon and in counseling is helpful. It is also exhausting. She finds that a commitment even to the smallest Kundalini Yoga practice helps recharge her physically, bolster her courage to speak her truth, and balance her emotions to create a neutral mind.

### EXERCISE
### FIGURE-EIGHT NECK ROLLS
An exercise this student found to be a life saver is also very simple.

1. Close your eyes. Begin to rotate your head in a figure-eight pattern.
2. Bring your chin all the way to your left shoulder; then rotate the chin forward along the collarbone until it reaches the center of the chest.
3. Then drop the head straight back, and rotate the head toward the right until the chin touches the right shoulder.
4. Once again press the chin along the collarbone until it reaches the center.
5. Then drop the head straight back, and rotate it toward the left until the chin again touches the left shoulder.
6. Continue to make your figure eights in a smooth, continuous movement, twenty-six times, working your way up to fifty-four times. Go slowly. Breathe through your nose, long and deep.

The key element of the exercise is that it is linked to the breath. Inhale when your chin touches the left shoulder, and exhale when your head touches the right shoulder. The movement is slow, and so is the breath.

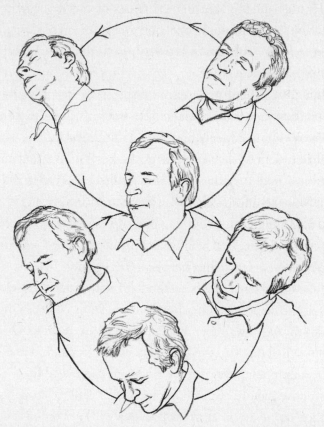

*Effects:* This exercise functions on a number of levels. It helps release muscle tension in the neck, which then takes more newly oxygenated blood to your brain, eyes, and ears. Your thyroid gets massaged and balanced; its brilliance brings a more youthful glow to your face.

If you want to take it one step further, step into the shower and let the water hit the areas under your arms and throughout your throat and across your heart area. Water and breath are great healers. Start with warm water and end with cold.

In the science of Kundalini Yoga and Meditation, breath patterns can do subtle and miraculous things for our body, mind, and soul. Since our brain is organized in hemispheres, any time we do a right/left focus on the breath, we are helping the neural pathways in our brain to connect across those hemispheres. Linking the movement and the breath help to super-oxygenate the blood. Counting the times of the movement becomes a mantra that takes your mind's attention away from all obsessive patternings.

The student with the marriage crisis often does this figure-eight movement before she goes into a counseling session with her husband. It takes only two or three minutes, and she finds that it really relaxes her and allows her to be fully present. This freeing up of the throat chakra is a simple way to get the connection going between the head and the heart, which is crucial to the process of healing our relationships. The exercise also opens the blood vessels to the brain, allowing newly oxygenated blood to flow in, giving greater clarity and insight.

I had a student once who had prayed very earnestly for her marriage to be healed. There had been many problems, most specifically a very troubled sexual relationship between the partners. When the marriage ended, she took this as proof that God did not exist. She discovered in the process of the divorce that her husband was homosexual. Divorce was, in her case, the only way for her marriage to be healed. Over time, she began to realize that her prayers had been answered, but as is so often the case, the answered prayer was not easy to recognize at first.

So many students are working to heal or find relationships. In developing their ability to speak the truth, they will find the peaceful, supportive relationships they long for, because they will be supportive of themselves first. Only when you are being true to yourself will you have the capacity to be true to another. Only when you love yourself will you fully receive the love of another and be able to give love fully in return.

**Begin your quest for your most authentic self. It is the surest path to happiness.**

If you deny parts of who you are and why you are here on earth, it will inevitably manifest itself in disease in the body. In thirty years of working with people, I have seen a devastating level of illness I believe results from people hiding from their own true nature.

Since hiding from ourselves is very common, there are consequently a great number of diseases that affect us in the throat chakra. Among the most common are dental problems, sore throats, loss of hearing, thyroid problems, and the one area of throat chakra disease that is epidemic in modern society, the disease of addiction.

Of course, there are many things to which people can be addicted, but I find it interesting that the most popular substance addictions—alcohol, cigarettes, food—come into our bodies through the area of the throat chakra. When I work with students who are conquering their addictions, I come from the perspective of someone who used to be an addict as well. I have been addicted to drugs and spent many years of my life that way. I can honestly say that coupled with my growing faith in God, Kundalini Yoga and Meditation are what helped me heal.

Sometimes when you are very low in energy, you feel like having bourbon on the rocks or black tea or a cigarette, whatever it is you are trying to avoid. You lose your willpower. Let's talk about what you can do as a substitute.

If you know breath of fire you are lucky, because that will revitalize you, but you may look odd doing it if you are in the marketplace. So instead, breathe in very deeply, wherever you are, hold as long as comfortable, and then breathe out. How many breaths does it take? Seven.

You'll find the increased oxygen giving you extra energy, and soon you'll move past your cravings.

**"If you can inhale and hold seven breaths, your oxygen will be completely circulated through your blood system, and you shall not need what you are longing to have."**

**—Yogi Bhajan**

The yogic teachings seem to dovetail with many other paths to recovery—therapy, religion, alternative healing practices. The variety of paths to healing that students take is kaleidoscopic. Whatever path you chose, Kundalini Yoga and Meditation only enhance whatever else you are doing to nurture yourself.

**Addictions become active when we are not living and developing our truth. Addictions are about hiding from the truth.**

When we "need" a drink or a smoke or some sugar, what we "need" is to avoid some truth we'd rather not deal with or speak about. In alcoholic families, the "saying" of what is going on, the naming of the truth of the situation, is the ultimate taboo. That is the importance for recovering addicts to be able to say, in a safe place, "I am an alcoholic." When we open our throat chakra and allow the talent of truth to flow freely, miracles happen.

**One shadow emotion of the fifth chakra is denial.**

Denial, or not being able to speak your truth, can be a valid coping and survival mechanism in our lives, but it is just that, a mechanism. It is not the way we are designed to live. People become patterned in their childhood. That pattern clouds their true identity as an adult.

**Humor is another tool that can release truth, because in order for something to be funny, it also has to be some kind of essential truth, usually a painful one.**

Going to a comedy club, renting a funny movie, reading a humorous book are great, fun things to do. They will also help heal your physical body. Of course, the healing power of humor is not a new idea, and there are many books devoted to this topic alone. The actual physical action of laughing causes you to breathe deeper; you have to breathe more fully into your lungs in order for your diaphragm to make the rapid movements that make up laughter. Sometimes I actually have students perform the physical act of laughing for a three-minute period. At first they resist and their laughing sounds phony and forced, but after about thirty seconds the sheer silliness of what they are doing usually catches up with them, and then I have a hard time getting them to stop.

Another easy way to begin to open the throat chakra is through the use of color. The color associated with this chakra is blue. I often tell students who are concentrating their self-healing efforts on the throat chakra to imagine a variety of blue things when they are meditating or just relaxing. It's very simple when you are lying in bed before you go to sleep to focus your mind on imagining various beautiful things in the color of blue: skies, an ocean, sapphires, aquamarines, blueberries, or whatever travels across your mind. I love to fill my windows with blue glass and see the sun shining through them.

When I'm feeling weak in this chakra, I almost always wear a pendant with a blue stone, a smoky aquamarine. I love to wear it on speaking engagements because it reminds me to speak truth. Wearing a particular color is a very subtle form of meditation, it reminds us of a quality of the spirit. Most traditional religious garb evolved this way. The clothes or adornments function as reminders of our spiritual path. Although most people in modern life don't have a religious dress code, we are certainly free to choose our clothes and and jewelry to help us with our healing and personal growth. It's easy to do and can be very effective. These small suggestions are effective because they are cumulative and because they are gifts of healing you give yourself.

I had a student who was a perfect example of how these very simple yogic practices can change your life. This student was an artist who had a number of throat chakra problems—strep throat, a car accident that damaged her neck, a lot of dental problems. She began doing a forty-day exercise and meditation to clear her throat chakra. She decided to wear a blue pendant and as much blue as she could during that period. She also made a pledge to sing in the shower, which she thought was silly, but agreed to try.

Like many urban dwellers, she had often worn black. The first thing that happened was that she almost instantly started getting compliments about how great she looked in blue. This gave her more confidence, and she began to feel as if she was healing. The blue she was wearing helped focus her attention on this part of her body and her new vision of a throat chakra that was overflowing with vitality.

Very shortly into the forty-day period, her chronic neck pain started to diminish. She also began to receive new inspiration about her work as an artist. As is often the case, the healing in her throat chakra was also affecting the chakras surrounding it. She was able to begin to tap into her sixth talent, the talent of intuition. Looking well and making great strides in her work all combined to make her feel better. She began to believe in the process she was undergoing, and that only deepened the healing.

She was also calmer and more relaxed because of her meditation and yoga. She enjoyed singing in the shower—that was just plain fun, and put a smile on that face of hers, which looked so pretty in all that blue. The result of all of these seemingly silly little things that took only fifteen or twenty minutes a day—all this culminated in her being pain-free and happier and more successful in her work by the end of the forty days. That was a far greater result than she had achieved with anything else she had tried.

Over and over again in teaching yoga and meditation, I have seen students begin to open their throat chakras, and who they really are emerges through their language and communication. Another easy way to begin to open this area is to begin to breathe consciously.

**Conscious breath is a huge part of the practice of Kundalini Yoga, and the simplest way to begin is to make an effort to breathe only through your nose.**

That sounds so simple as to not even be worth your time, but it can make almost instantaneous improvements in your health. Your personal breathing apparatus is designed so that you should breathe almost exclusively through your nose. Your nose is an intricate and ingenious air filtering system. Very often when people get stressed, breathing through their nose is one of the first things to go.

Generally, breathing through your mouth is a panic response. When you begin to do that, you trigger the production of endorphins, which tell your body that the crisis is real. Simply by focusing on breathing through your nose, even at the gym or when you are running or walking, you will begin to decrease your body's unneeded production of endorphins, automatically making you feel less stressed out.

Of course, there are many more things you could do than just these small things to begin opening up your speaking powers, but I have great reverence for small actions, and here is why. Our various chakras become out of balance because of small daily abuses, and they will be most completely healed with small daily gestures of caring. Every time in your life that someone told you to "shut up" closed off a piece of your throat chakra. With every cleansing breath you consciously take through your nose, a part of your throat chakra begins to open up and heal.

Many people come to me who are deep in their addictions. Students on the way to their cars will light up a cigarette after doing a yoga class, and I would never tell them to do any differently, which often surprises people.

It has been my experience that the more you do this work, every day clearing away those small bits of damage, eventually, your body will join your mind and spirit in realizing that the craving itself is an illusion, the craving is a systematic error in your biochemistry that developed as a child, as a way to avoid truths you mistakenly thought you couldn't handle. Your body will come out of denial and into truth. Addiction is the separation of you and your soul. The separation is so painful, you could die from the pain. So you fill that space with an addiction until you are shown a way to bring your body and your soul as one.

Students who have had problems with food cravings, after beginning the practice of Kundalini Yoga and Meditation, begin choosing more healthy foods, more fresh vegetables, more fresh fruits, more whole foods, less meat, fish, chicken, and eggs. I have many students who have come to me with all manner of eating disorders. Without exception, those who continue even the smallest form of practice have had significant healing.

There are a number of scientific reasons why this may be true. The main one may be that almost every exercise done in the practice of Kundalini Yoga is done with the eyes closed and the focus of the eyes rolled up to the third eye, the area between the eyebrows. This is the location of the pituitary gland, the gland that regulates serotonin. And serotonin, of course, has a large role in regulating our appetite.

Humans love to find out the mechanical, scientific reason that something works. I find it fascinating, too, but the more profound reason these students experience such remarkable healing in the area of eating disorders has to do with the opening of the throat chakra.

I have a student who is a renowned and gifted psychotherapist. She has a real talent for pinpointing exactly where a certain behavioral pattern comes from in someone else's childhood, and even in her own life. She acknowledges that finding out how a problem started doesn't necessarily lead to the solution. She often comes to me and asks for a specific exercise or meditation to heal a certain emotional pattern. My therapist friend has discovered that doing a meditation for an eating disorder she knows is rooted in her patient's childhood is far more effective than analyzing exactly when, why, and how the disorder began.

When it comes to sculpting our bodies physically, I am sure that there are many choices out there, including liposuction, that will give us a more "perfect" body. If that is truly what you seek, you would be best to look elsewhere than to Kundalini Yoga and Meditation. The most profound change I have seen in my students, particularly those who suffer from distorted body image, is that doing this work not only improves their body, but makes them love their bodies exactly as they are.

I know how easy it is to develop a negative body self-image. In my teens I abused diet drugs, and to this day if I am feeling down on myself, I look in the mirror and see a fat person staring back.

As women in America, we are surrounded by images that assault us, telling us repeatedly that our bodies are inadequate. People spend millions of dollars trying to achieve an ideal that is unnatural and unhealthy.

When you start loving your body with the practice of Kundalini Yoga, when you detach from these false magazine images and see what a miracle machine your body is, it is just then that you most often find that your body begins to become ideal—your *own* ideal body, not someone else's falsely imposed image of an ideal body.

When I teach a yoga set, I don't tell the students a certain exercise will give them "killer abs" or "buns of steel." In a sense, every yoga exercise is for your whole body. You may have noticed that your body comes in one piece. We do not live in Lego Land, and we don't practice yoga as though our bodies were composed of a lot of separate parts, some more inferior or valuable than others. The real tangible result is, we begin to like and appreciate our bodies more, and they become healthier and stronger.

When you start to create your practice, your program of yoga and meditation, you will begin craving the foods that will be most healing to you, and they will taste so delicious. You will find yourself going to the fresh fruit and veggie aisle. And, of course, yogi tea. I've seen it happen time and time again.

**A healthy diet does include treats; it's all a matter of balance.**

Part of the challenge of healing and growing is finding balance. It's fitting, because the physical location in our bodies of this talent includes the neck, which is a miracle of balance we almost never think about. When you watch a new baby trying to hold its head up, you can see what a circus act this simple action really is. Metaphorically, keeping the balance between our head and our heart is one of the most important factors in the quality of our lives. That balance is called compassion and kindness. It hurts our heart and the hearts of others when we carelessly go around letting our Monkey Mind speak for us.

A student of mine had a grandmother who was in her nineties. She moved into a retirement apartment with twenty-four-hour nursing care, which was a difficult adjustment for her. It was a good solution, though, because it still provided her with independence.

When her grandson first came to visit her at the apartment, she proudly showed him her gas range. She told him that she would never agree to move to an apartment with an electric range, she'd always cooked with gas, and she refused to move in until they put in the gas burners. When he looked at the stove he saw that there were electric burners, but didn't say a thing. She prepared him lunch, cooking on the electric burners and chattering happily about the convenience of cooking with gas. Now, this student is someone I know to be very particular about details, and yet he had the wisdom to let his nana cook on her "gas" stove without distraction.

**The truth is more important than the mere facts of the thing. That is truth in action.**

Incorporating yoga as a physical and spiritual practice in your life will help you heal your soul, using your body as the tool for that healing. And it's a reciprocal relationship, because when your body heals, your mind heals and your soul heals. They are interrelated.

If neck aches, dental problems, sore throats, hearing problems, thyroid problems, or addictions have had an impact on your life, this is your body telling you that there is an imbalance going on, using the only language it has to warn you, the language of pain and disease. It's not just heredity or toxic conditions that cause these diseases. They are directly related to the need of your soul to cry out its truth. Your soul longs for truth, and using the science of Kundalini Yoga and Meditation, your body can help lead you to its discovery.

## FIFTH CHAKRA EXERCISES
## EXERCISE FOR YOUTH AND REJUVENATION

1. Stand with a straight spine.
2. Clasp the hands together in front of the chest, extending the index fingers. Keep the elbows relaxed down by the sides.
3. Inhale deeply through the nose, and extend the arms up and back over the head as you lean the body back at a sixty-degree angle. Drop the head back, putting a stretch on the throat. Keep the hands clasped together as you lean back.
4. Exhale through the nose as you return to the original position.
5. Breathe powerfully.

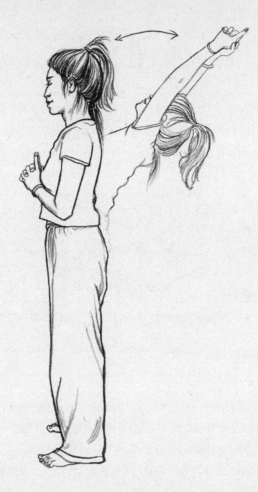

*Effects:* This exercise powerfully stimulates the thyroid and parathyroid, the guardians of your health and beauty. Improper balance of these two glands can make you age before your time. The skin, the complexion, and the outward appearance are affected by the thyroid.

## MEDITATION FOR BREAKING HABITS

1. Sit in a comfortable pose. Keep the spine and especially the first six lower vertebrae locked straight.
2. Make the hands into fists and extend the thumbs out straight.
3. Place the pads of the thumbs on the temples at the sides of the forehead, and find the niche where the thumbs just fit in perfectly.

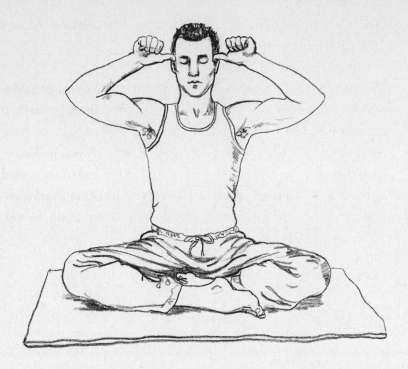

4.   Lock the back molars together and keep the lips closed.

5.   Alternately press the molars together and then release, just like when you are biting down. You will feel a muscle moving in rhythm directly under your thumbs. Keep a firm pressure on the temples with the thumb pads.

6.   The eyes are closed and turned up, looking toward the third eye point.

7.   With each pressure on the molars, silently vibrate the sounds "Sa-Ta-Na-Ma" at the brow.

8.   Continue five to seven minutes, breathing long and deeply through your nose. With practice, the time can be increased up to thirty-one minutes.

*Effects:* In modern-day society we are addicted to many things, from smoking to eating, drinking, or drugs; and on a more mental level we are often addicted to acceptance, emotional love, and even to thinking! All of these lead us to insecurity in our behavior and choices.

> This meditation is used as a remedy for all kinds of physical and mental addictions. The pressure from the thumbs exerts a current into the central part of the brain. An imbalance here makes mental and physical addictions seemingly unbreakable. This meditation will correct this central brain imbalance, and is especially helpful for someone who is attempting to rehabilitate from drug dependence, mental illness, overeating, as well as phobic conditions.

# 6

# The Sixth Chakra

INTUITION

"As human beings we were not given claws, thorns, or hooves to shield ourselves. Instead the Creator gave us the ability to develop our intuition for protection."

—Yogi Bhajan

The human talent of intuition is located in the sixth chakra, generally defined as the area at our brow point. In the classical chakra system, it is related to the point between the eyebrows, sometimes referred to as the third eye point. This area is where the pituitary gland, also known as the master gland, is located. It is the pituitary that is responsible for the secretion of serotonin, which recent research has pinpointed as being a major factor in the health of our emotional lives. The human talent of intuition is the receiving end of our connection with God.

**"Your intelligence should flow through your chakras under the supervision of your intuition. It is a simple science, through which you will become successful in life."**

**—Yogi Bhajan**

Most of the meditations are done with our eyes closed. We ask the students to imagine they are looking upward and in, as though they were focusing their gaze through this third eye point. Even if you aren't using any formal meditation, the very act of closing your eyes and letting your eyes focus in this way can have a tremendously relaxing effect.

**"To control your emotions you have to concentrate on the sixth center."**

**—Yogi Bhajan**

MEDITATION ON YOUR THIRD EYE POINT
To develop intuition and your higher powers to experience your third eye:

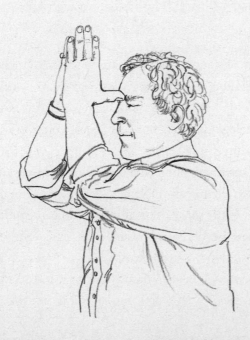

1.  Place your thumbs on the space between your eyebrows.
2.  Press firmly and roll the eyes up to where you are pressing with your eyelids down.
3.  Do this for three minutes. Keep your breath long and deep, and with every inhale and exhale, feel the breath going in and out of this point on your forehead.
4.  After three minutes, release your thumbs and sit quietly with your hands in your lap, eyes rolled up and focused at the middle of the forehead. As you inhale, mentally vibrate the word "Sat," and as you exhale, mentally vibrate the word "Nam." Continue for another three minutes.
5.  Inhale and relax. Then open your eyes, slowly look around, and relax.

*Effects*: Usually after a brief period you will begin to see colors or patterns of light. Often after you have settled into the practice you will begin to see an amazing indigo blue color, and this is the exact color classically associated with this chakra.

**"If you are conscious, you are alert, and you are intuitive, there is no place for error."**

**—Yogi Bhajan**

When I hear of people going broke because they have spent thousands of dollars calling "psychic hot lines," my heart is so sad for them. It is their own "psychic hot line" for which they are searching. Fortunately, tapping into your own psychic hot line is not going to cost you $3.99 a minute. It is absolutely free.

Our psychic hot line is our intuition, which is the receiving end of our connection to God. Within the spiritual design of our bodies, we receive God's word through the sense of intuition. What we refer to in yoga as the third eye point goes beyond our physical eyes. This third eye gives us our depth and dimension in the subtle worlds. It is the energy center where we can master the flow and sense of duality in our mind. For example, if our intellectual mind gives us a yes to some question, our intuitive sense may say no. If we could master the sixth chakra, we would never be confused by the various polarities in life and would be able to read between the lines, so to speak, with this third eye. This is true intuition.

In his wonderful book, *How Do We Know When It's God?* Dan Wakefield addresses exactly this question. He talks in his book about how the practice of yoga helped enhance his growing Christian faith during a time of crisis. He says, "In going to yoga, in trying to pray through the flesh rather than words, I feel like I am going back to basics, going back to the body to find the spirit."

Here, in the sixth chakra, we are beginning to move into the higher realms of intellect and spirituality. That is why, for the sixth chakra, there is no corresponding element. In the last three chakras—the sixth, seventh, and eighth—we are now moving into thought and spirit.

**Confusion is the shadow emotion of the human talent of intuition.**

Recently when I was teaching, a man in the front of the class began to distract my attention. As he did each of the poses, his facial expressions became tremendously distorted, much more so than I was used to seeing even from those students who come from the "grunt and grind" school of weight lifting. I spoke to this student after class and asked him why he made these expressions. He confessed to me he had been feeling as if his brain was "out of control" and that there was a "constant stream of chatter" that was making him feel confused and depressed.

I sensed that he, like a lot of people who suffer from depression, was probably a very intuitive person. Since he didn't have the tools to cultivate his intuition, he became confused, which leads to depression. What was happening to this man happens to so many of us. Certainly, judging by the widespread use of antidepressants, this is a problem that plagues millions.

**"You will be tested—but that is the nature of life.**
**When life is very rough, be very calm.**

Go inside and find your soul.

Be neutral and meditative, and the way will become more
  clear."

—Yogi Bhajan

The three-minute exercise I gave him is deceptively simple, and I
challenged him to try it for forty days, not missing a single day.

EXERCISE TO FREE YOU FROM CONFUSION
AND DEPRESSION

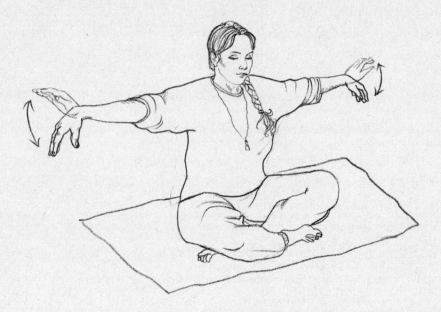

1.    Sit quietly on the floor with your legs crossed.

2.    Extend your arms straight out to the sides like great wings, palms
flat and facing the floor.

3.    Begin flapping just your wrists and hands rapidly, as though you
were flying furiously through the air.

4.    Your arms will move slightly from the shoulders, but the action is in
the wrists.

5.    Breathe in long, deep inhales and exhales.

6.    Do this motion for three minutes.

*Effects:* Although it sounds easy, it does get tiring and painful, but he did it! He persevered and did it every single day for forty days without exception, and continues to do it every day. The change I saw in him was remarkable. His depression and confusion began to lift, and now when he sits in front of me in class, I see a totally different person, a quiet, happy face.

It doesn't mean that his troubles are over, but using this one tool has led him to other tools. He is on his way to a daily spiritual practice, God willing, for the rest of his life. That will give him a healthier, happier life.

**Intuition whispers to us in many ways; one of the most important ways it speaks to us is through the language of dreams and metaphors.**

**"Go inside and listen to your inner voice.**
**Every question has an answer.**
**Your soul is full of wisdom and knows the way."**

**—Yogi Bhajan**

I often practice using my intuition in very simple ways, for example, while I am driving. Before I head off somewhere, I take the time prayerfully to consider the various routes I might take, and see which one intuitively hits me. I started doing this as a way of using my intuition to avoid traffic jams, but I find it provides me with even more. Oftentimes, when I make this prayerful intention about what route to take, I am inspired by something that I see along the way. Sometimes the results are merely pleasant; other times they are profound and life-changing.

**If you can't see God in all, you can't see God at all.**

One day I was driving along Sunset Boulevard, the route toward which my intuition had guided me. On that particular day, I was feeling a little disheartened about my teaching, wondering if these teachings were being heard and what more I could do to make sure they were being received. I started questioning if people were really ready to commit to new ways of thinking and being, or were we stuck in our addictive patterns as a society.

These thoughts were rambling through my mind. Just at that moment, I looked up to that old famous hotel, the Chateau Marmont, to the balcony of the penthouse where I used to teach private clients who lived in that hotel. A few days a week, I would come to their suite and take them through their yoga practice on that very balcony. We always faced toward the east, toward the morning sun and also toward an enormous three-story billboard featuring the Marlboro Man. I remembered that we had always laughed at the irony of the fact that we were doing yoga in front of a gigantic cigarette.

On this particular day, as I was driving down Sunset, I looked up at what I thought was the Marlboro billboard. As luck would have it, traffic was stuck. I looked closer at the billboard and realized that it was not a cigarette ad, but an anti-smoking ad. It had the Marlboro man all right, and he was smoking, but the cigarette was drooping. The message at the bottom of the billboard was that smoking is a leading cause of impotence. I burst into laughter as I realized what I was seeing. That giant cigarette in front of which I had done hours of yoga had wilted. I almost felt as if we had wilted it ourselves with the power of our practice.

More important, on a metaphorical level, I felt the billboard had an intuitive message for me. The message was that people were in fact ready to make positive changes in their lives and health. That billboard existed because the voters of California had passed a proposition that allowed tax money to be used to create anti-smoking campaigns.

Thirty years ago, when I started teaching yoga, that would have been unthinkable. Things really are changing, and I felt that I had on some small level been a part of that change. I felt intuitively I would get to be a bigger part of that change as time went on.

**"If you need an answer to something, just concentrate.**
**In one second the answer will come to you.**

**It's a law of the Universal Mind.**

**The Universal Mind is always there to feed you.**

**Right within you there is a very feeble, simple, unoffending, absolutely knowledgeable, little conscious voice. It talks. It's not loud. It's very soft."**

—Yogi Bhajan

Not very long after I had my "intuitive drive" down Sunset, I was approached by a dear yoga student about writing a book. After months of work, the proposal was accepted. This is the book you are reading now. In a way, I credit all of that happening to my willingness to be intuitive about such a small daily thing as which way I should drive to Santa Monica. If I hadn't listened to my intuition and driven down Sunset, a route I don't like very much, I would never have noticed that billboard. The billboard was the answer to my prayer, "Can the world hear these ancient teachings?" I realized that if you can't see God in all, you can't see God at all. God lives even in the Marlboro Man.

**If you open yourself to your intuition in small ways, the really big messages will find a way through.**

Sometimes the message doesn't come to you right away. I have often bought a book on impulse, read some of it, decided that it didn't appeal to me, and put it on the shelf, only to happen upon it later to find that I was now ready to hear whatever that book had to tell me. Your intuition can send you messages you are not ready to hear. This is very good news, because it means that intuition is not a make-or-break deal. We don't have to worry that if we don't get the message the first time, it will be lost forever.

**When we are balanced within ourselves, then we can do the will of God.**

One student has experienced a tremendous upsurge in her own ability to intuit since she has begun a serious practice of yoga and meditation. She is a highly creative and famous musician. Although she is intuitive in her art, she has begun to be more intuitive in her life, with dramatic results.

Recently, she was on the road, riding in a tour bus late at night. The bus slowed down, and she became aware that there was a traffic accident up ahead. She suddenly became seized with the desire to help. She rushed out of the bus. With a number of surprised onlookers watching, she was able to lift up one of the bent and broken vehicles, freeing a passenger who had been trapped inside. When the incident had passed, she didn't recall rationally making the decision to do it; her intuition merely called her up, and her body willingly complied.

She had acted from the place between the negative mind and the positive mind. The negative mind is the mind that says, "I can't," and the positive mind is the mind that says, "I can." Yogis refer to this in-between place as the "neutral mind," or the non-reactionary mind, or the intuitive mind. If she had stopped for an instant to think "I can," that would have been matched by her negative mind with "I can't." She acted, as we would say yogically, "beyond time and space."

I have heard stories like this over the years—mothers who lifted cars off their children—but I had never been privileged to speak to someone to whom this had actually happened. When I spoke with her, she seemed very humbled by it. She had no sense of having done it at all. When we are most open to the call of God, it is in those moments that it is clearly demonstrated to us that we are not the "doer." God is the Doer, and when we are balanced within ourselves, it is then we can truly do the will of God. It's no surprise to me that the pure will of God brings one miracle after another into our lives.

This is where the wisdom begins, when we enter the realm of seeing things as neither good nor bad.

**Real, true intuition, almost nine times out of ten, is the intuition of joy.**

The fact I ended up making yoga my life's work was a most blessed good fortune. My journey to yoga began in the sixties when I was a flower child in San Francisco. I was a seeker of truth. I had spent time living in a Zen Buddhist center on Maui, in Hawaii, and I had been accepted into the Buddhist nunnery in Kamakura, Japan. This was in 1969. I had returned to the mainland briefly before I was to head to Japan when I ran into an old dear friend, Marky J. He lived in Carmel Valley, California, where his father was the village minister. Everyone there knew him, for he had spent his whole life in the Valley. While I was dressed in bell-bottoms, an Indian madras shirt, with lots of beads and wild, bushy hair, he looked straight as an arrow, with his saddle shoes, button-down collar, short, combed blond hair, and thick, black-rimmed glasses. In his low, slow, drawling voice, he invited me to his twenty-first birthday party. After the party at his mother's house, we were alone, and he asked me to meditate with him that late January night. After the meditation, as we opened our eyes, he told me that in three days he would drive me to Tucson, where he was to leave me at an ashram. He said God had told him he was to take me there.

I asked him, "What is an ashram?" He said, "It is a place to pray, meditate, do yoga, and serve people." I answered that yes, I would be ready in three days. I didn't think about it, I simply followed my intuition and said yes.

After our road trip of five days, made in a VW bug, Marky J., his big white German shepherd, and I arrived in Tucson. My friend pulled up to a big house that was being used as an ashram and a yoga center. He stayed for seven days and meditated. Then he paid my first month's rent, which was seventy-five dollars for room and board, and on the eighth day he left me there. To this day I have not seen him again. Who was he? My spirit guide? My angel? We all have them, we really do.

If I had been rational or practical, which most of my life I have not, I would have said no back in Carmel Valley on that cold January night. I would have thought to myself, "This doesn't make sense, I'll pass on this." Just like my musician friend who lifted the car without a thought, I said, "Yes, I'll go." I believe you have to follow these intuitive hunches, or else you will become one of those people who is always saying, "I *knew* I should have done that, but I didn't trust myself." Or you might end up saying, "I just *knew* what was going to happen, but I didn't say anything." Follow your intuition and your dreams.

When I took my first yoga class, I cried my way through it. Something opened up inside of me, and I felt I had finally come home. I knew this would become my life's work, and I knew I had been longing for this; I had such a longing to belong. When I was a child my parents called me "Mary-Sit-and-Do-Nothing." I can only imagine that this was because I was a born meditator, and back when I was a child that was translated into sitting and doing nothing.

As a child I did not speak well, and at the age of five they had me tested to see if I had a mental imbalance. I loved to be creative, and I remember playing Mary in the Easter pageant at church every year, exclaiming, "He has arisen, he has arisen!" So my love of God was part of me even then. There are clues to who we become in our childhood, and it's important to remember them. I always loved to grow my hair long, and then joined a religion where our practice is to never cut our hair, but to wind it up on top of our head, and then wrap it in a turban. I had a destiny, as we all do, and it began to whisper itself to me through intuition.

The things we love, the things that attract us are like signposts along the way. Every one of us has these signposts, which constantly appear to us. I urge you to look for them, and if you are a parent, to watch for them in your children, so that you might better understand who they are, and guide them in the right direction with helpful tools.

**If you love a thing, if you completely lose track of time when you are doing it, that is something you are meant to do.**

Sometimes, for the cynical, this intuitive call is covered in sarcasm. The call does not come in a sarcastic way, but sarcasm is used to avoid hearing it. I have a student who is a stand-up comic, and for years she used to watch stand-up comics and ridicule how bad they were, and yet she couldn't stop watching them. She was so attracted to the art form she claimed to hate. This student credits her study of yoga as part of what gave her the courage to write five minutes of material and throw herself onstage, and she loved it and has been loving it ever since. Clearly it is what she was meant to do, as she is now a working professional comic.

**Yoga is such an invaluable tool in developing intuition, because each exercise or meditation allows us to run a little practice drill with our body, mind, and spirit.**

There are many yoga exercises or meditations that seem pointless, boring, or irritating, and that is just exactly their point. By committing to the exercise for three minutes, or even seven minutes, you are agreeing to go on a little journey. As you journey through discomfort, irritation, or deep-seated emotions, as you move past these things, using your breath, you can begin to hear messages from your intuitive self.

**Experiencing the struggle, even for a few minutes, will set you free.**

The everyday static of irritation or discomfort is cleared away by experiencing it intensely in a yoga exercise. You can begin to see the irritation or discomfort for the illusion that it is. Without a practice that allows us to focus on feeling discomfort in a safe way, we can get trapped in living our whole lives running away from discomfort. So many of the messages we get in this society are about eliminating the uncomfortable, the awkward, the irritating.

We are bombarded thousands of times a day with the drumbeat of "Get a new car, a new outfit, a new perfume, and everything will be okay." The purchase of each of these objects promises to make us more comfortable, more happy, more loved, more admired. There is no advertising slogan that tells us to experience fully the irritation or annoyance, or God forbid, pain. Pain is as much a gift as joy, and that is something our culture does not value. If we experience that everything comes from God, we welcome each new day as a new adventure.

Yoga allows you to focus for a few minutes on what you have spent the entire day running away from, see it for the paper tiger it is, and get on with your day and your life. Once you have focused intensely on that pain or irritation, your mind is almost miraculously quieted down. Once your mind is quieted down, the "radio frequency" of your intuition begins to speak to you loudly and clearly.

I know with every cell in my body that doing yoga and meditation will help you to fulfill your life's purpose—the call of your soul. Even the students who don't make complete shifts in their life plan often commit to a deeper, more challenging version of their lives.

I have seen students leave highly paid jobs, take a financial gamble, and pursue work that their intuition tells them is what they are meant to be doing. I have seen them challenged, and make serious downshifts in their material lifestyle. Now, you may be reading this and thinking, "That sounds terrible." I won't lie to you and say that these transitions have been pain-free, but I can say without exception that the students who have chosen this challenging path have ended up being among the happiest people I have known. I have seen other students follow their intuitive, creative selves and gain great prosperity.

> **"Going through life without intuition is like driving a car which has no side mirror and no rearview mirror. All you can see is just straight ahead."**
>
> **—Yogi Bhajan**

There is a student who was very successful in a career in which his job was to evaluate and criticize the work of writers. He was good at it, and he made a lot of money, but he had a gnawing feeling that he was wasting his life. He always used to say, "Well I'm not getting any younger." That had become his mantra. He nursed a low-grade depression, overate, and drank too much, but was to the outside world a very successful guy.

This man found his way to my class. He tells me now that even after taking a class, he thought it was "a complete waste of time, a lot of hippie mumbo jumbo." After that evaluation I can't imagine why he came back, but he did. He made time in his busy executive schedule for something he had determined was a complete waste of time. He became a committed student, coming to class regularly a couple of times a week.

He began making changes in his life. He got sober, he started considering the possibility he was doing the wrong job. Instead of criticizing writers, maybe he should become one. When I asked him recently why he started to recognize this, he did not have an answer. I think what was happening to this man, almost unconsciously, was that doing yoga and meditation allowed him to begin listening to his intuition, which he had been ignoring all along.

Ultimately, this man quit his secure executive position and began trying to form a career for himself as a writer. It was not easy or instant, but ultimately he has become a successful working writer, and is happy in a way he never dreamt possible.

When I spoke with him about this transition, he said he felt that doing yoga was really the first step toward this life change. He says, "The yoga came first, and I worked hard at it, and a lot of the time I hated it, but I kept coming back. And then I started taking a look at my drinking, and I decided to get sober. Then I rediscovered my connection to Judaism. I quit my job and started doing what I'm doing now, and I am so grateful for all of these changes. But I think it was really the yoga that kick-started me."

That student's story is typical of what I see happen to people when they get started on the path of yoga and meditation. The science of Kundalini Yoga states there is knowledge and awareness in every cell of your body. All of the platitudes in the world won't wake up the intuition your body has on a cellular level. All of you exists in each and every cell of your body, and this ancient science of yoga is specifically designed to wake you up on a cellular level.

**Your body speaks to you metaphorically through the language of disease.**

Part of this inherent wisdom in our bodies is seen in the creation of disease. One of the Kundalini Yoga students recently told me a remarkable story. This young woman, who had just turned thirty, was trapped in a job that had brought her material success but no real satisfaction. Her boss was both abusive and very dependent on her. She felt as if she poured all her energy into him and got nothing back. Her feelings about him were vague and unformed. She couldn't even connect that what was wrong with her might be that she was in the wrong job.

She started getting migraines and took medication for them, which helped somewhat. She still didn't take stock of her life choices in any way. Then a very disturbing thing happened. She started lactating—milk started flowing from her breasts—and yet she was childless and had never been pregnant. When she went to the doctors, a non-malignant tumor was discovered on her pituitary gland, her third eye point, the home of her intuition.

She left her job. During that time off, as she prepared for surgery, she began to take a deeper look at her life and the way she was living. She had surgery to have the tumor removed, and it was successful.

While she was still in the hospital, a friend gave her a book on Kundalini Yoga, which talked about the third eye point and intuition, the exact area where her tumor had grown. After that, she started a very rigorous Kundalini Yoga practice, taking her to a much healthier weight. She is a remarkably different person. She left the profession she was in and began a new and very rewarding career in another area to which she had always felt attracted but had never had the courage to try. Although she had been physically active before she began yoga, she lost twenty pounds after she started her practice.

She was an extremely diligent student. A few months into her practice of yoga and meditation, her headaches disappeared. The tumor has never grown back, and she has stopped lactating. This student felt her intuition call out to her and ultimately use some mighty dramatic methods to get her attention. She found it ironic that her body actually began lactating when she was giving all her nurturing energies toward an abusive boss. Your body speaks to you metaphorically through the language of disease.

This student's enthusiasm for her yoga practice is infectious. In addition to the fact that she has had amazing improvements in her life and health, she feels there have been other, more subtle benefits. She and her husband are both devoted yoga students. They do their yoga together at the beginning of their day. She feels that it has enhanced their intimacy as a couple, and has made them more patient and loving.

Kundalini Yoga and Meditation will help you develop intuition. After a while, your intuition doesn't have to be quite so showy to get your attention. As you begin to trust it more and more, it can speak to you in a less dramatic fashion and you will pay attention, because you know this talent to be real. Intuition is not a special talent available only to a gifted few, it is available to everyone who is willing to listen to themselves. When you think about how much we listen to messages that come from the outside world, you realize it makes sense to give at least equal credence to the messages that come from within us.

"Intuition is the real power. You all have it.
It is God's given gift."

—Yogi Bhajan

Oftentimes I connect with my intuition when I am looking for inspiration, especially on a creative project. I have found that a good way to kick-start this is being creative in ways that seem less high-stakes than whatever project I am contemplating. For example, when I want to decorate a room in my home or at the yoga center, I explore the creative possibilities of that room intuitively. Recently I did this by buying lots of fresh flowers of different colors from different parts of the world, from tropical to traditional. One week, I had blue flowers, one week red, one week yellow, and I felt the various moods of those colors in that room. When I at last spent the money on a red Oriental carpet, I knew it was a "red room."

If you were to deduce from the record number of antidepressants taken in Western society, you would have to conclude that we are in a depression epidemic. In some ways this is true, but I don't find this depressing. I think these statistics result partly from the fact people are more willing to admit they feel depressed. When I was growing up, it was simply never discussed.

**Yoga and meditation have been scientifically proven to increase the amount of serotonin and beta endorphins in the bloodstream.**

Though I do think the whole class of such serotonin reuptake inhibitor drugs as Prozac or Zoloft can be lifesavers for some people, Kundalini Yoga and Meditation will aid greatly in this healing process, whether done with antidepressant medication or on its own. In her fascinating book *Potatoes, Not Prozac*, Dr. Kathleen DesMaisons talks about how yoga and meditation have been scientifically proven to increase the amount of serotonin and beta endorphins in the bloodstream. Although I am not a clinical doctor, I know this to be true from my own teaching. I have seen many students eventually wean themselves from pharmaceuticals.

BOWING EXERCISE

This is a yoga exercise amazingly powerful for alleviating depression and enhancing intuition. Although it is one of the easiest exercises in Kundalini Yoga, it's highly effective.

1.   Sit comfortably, preferably on your heels in a kneeling position. If that is difficult, you can do it with your legs crossed in easy pose, or whatever

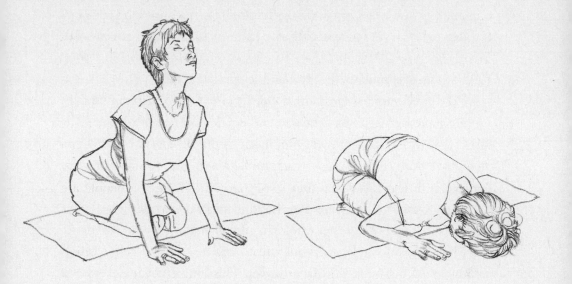

version works for you. Some students like to use a pillow to cushion their knees when they are kneeling.

2.  Place both palms on the floor and bow your head until your third eye point, the area between your eyebrows, touches the floor.

3.  Raise back up to the original position.

4.  Continue the bowing motion, lightly touching your forehead to the floor each time, keeping the neck and the spine relaxed and fluid.

5.  Your buttocks stay on your heels, both while bowing down and coming back up.

6.  Chant silently or aloud "Sat" as you come up, and "Nam" as you go down. Your eyes are closed and focused upward to the third eye point. The breath is long and slow through your nose. If you choose to chant silently, inhale your head up, exhale your head down.

*Effects:* Bowing is a part of almost every culture on earth, because it awakens the subtlety in us. We feel its effects even after doing it for just a short period of time. This is a great exercise to try for a longer period, but when done even for three minutes, it is wonderfully relaxing and elevating.

Bowing flexes the spine gently, loosens the neck muscles, engages the leg and arm muscles as well as all the muscles at the navel point. Finally, the upward focus of the eyes as well as the gentle touching of the third eye point stimulates the sixth and seventh chakras.

On a metaphorical level, the act of bowing represents many things. Some people feel it subjugates them to the will of someone or something else. However, in truth, bowing is honoring yourself and the divine creative force that lives within. It is a humble act, but all too often people confuse humility and humiliation.

Humility means understanding that you are a worthwhile and valuable person who is part of a greater whole. In great thankfulness and awe do we bow. Humiliation is giving up our will to another human being, falsely assuming that person is our higher power. This simple bowing exercise is good for your body and also serves as a physical reminder of our place in the whole vastness of creation. That's a lot to be going on in one little bow!

To me, the fact that one simple exercise can mean and do so much is part of what makes this ancient practice of yoga such a miracle. It seems perfectly natural that medical science is just beginning to discover and record what people have known for thousands of years. This yoga works; it can be a valuable tool in healing your body, your mind and your spirit.

To the skeptic who may be reading this, I say just try it, even one exercise, for just three minutes. See if you don't feel better.

**I've taught thousands of people yoga over the years, and I have never had anyone say the experience left him or her feeling nothing.**

Not everyone continues to practice Kundalini Yoga and Meditation. Most of the time when I ask students why they stopped, they didn't feel they had the time, or they weren't sure they were getting "a good enough workout." What I find most intriguing is many times people will come just to one class, and then go away, only to return years later and become extremely devoted practitioners of Kundalini Yoga. It's almost as though a seed was planted in them; something about the experience just stayed with them.

Do this one bowing exercise. If you begin and keep up, you will be kept up. If you choose to do this one exercise for three minutes or more a day for forty days, you will find that your depression will be far less severe. It doesn't mean you won't have down days, but it is a way to engage your body and all its resources so the down days become the exception rather than the rule.

I had a student who came to me when she was still in college, who had suffered from severe depression all her life. Many times she had contemplated suicide, and she came from a family where there had been a number of suicide deaths. She began her practice of yoga almost a decade ago. Early on in her practice she saw huge improvements in her ability to function and her well-being and happiness.

Eventually she ended up going into therapy. After much consideration, she began taking antidepressants. She maintains a faithful yoga practice and believes that both the medication and her yoga allow her to lead a normal, happy life. As she puts it, "I believe I have chronic clinical depression which needs medication, but I never would have been able to see that truth about myself if it had not been for my yoga practice. Doing yoga allowed the fog of gloom to clear enough for me to be able to rationally evaluate what I needed."

For this student and others, having yoga and meditation be part of her plan for overall health makes her a partner in her own healing. She doesn't just "take something" that makes her feel better, she "does something" that makes her feel better.

**It is essential you be an active participant in the creation of your own good mental health.**

## MEDITATION TO HEAL DEPRESSION

**I was taught a very powerful meditation to heal depression years ago by my teacher Yogi Bhajan. It is a little more complicated because it does involve the use of a mantra, but it yields such amazing results, I wanted to include it.**

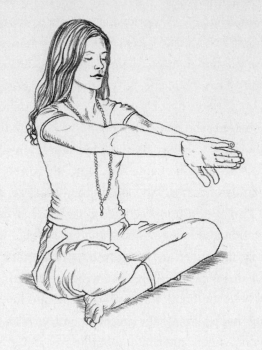

1.   Begin by sitting in a comfortable, cross-legged position.

2.   Extend your arms straight out in front of you, so the elbows are straight and the arms are parallel to the ground.

3.   Place the hands together back-to-back, so all the knuckles are touching and the thumbs are facing down.

4.   Close your eyes until they are only one-tenth open, so that just a little sliver of light comes through. Stare at the tip of your nose.

5.   Inhale very deeply, and on the exhale chant in a monotone the ancient sounds "Wah-Hey Gur-Roo." (This is a phonetic spelling. The closest translation of these sounds that would be familiar to us in the West is "Hallelujah—God Is Great Beyond Words.")

6.   Chant this as many times as you possibly can on one breath, eventually working your way up to saying the words sixteen times per each breath.

7.   Do this meditation at least three minutes, but make it your goal to increase it by a minute a day until you are able to do it for eleven minutes.

*Effects:* Focusing your eyes this way is something children love to do as a game. Just this eye focus alone can be incredibly calming. Chanting is similar to how acupuncture works. In acupuncture, you stimulate certain nerve clusters with needles, and thus effect change in other areas of the body.

If the chanting (the mantra) and the hand position (the mudra) seem overwhelming for you at this point, that's okay.

Begin more simply by just taking three minutes to close your eyes until they are only one-tenth open, and then focus your gaze at the tip of your nose. It may be somewhat blurry, and after a while it begins to be fun to focus on the way the images and the light blur and flicker.

I love to do this one when I am in line at the bank or the post office. It is almost instantly relaxing and allows me to keep shuffling along, keeping my place in line. I find I like being in line more if I use the time to mellow out with this eye exercise. Sometimes I feel so refreshed by the time I get to the front of the line that I find myself actually wishing the line were a little longer. To me nothing could be more powerful proof of the miracle of yogic meditation than this.

Since I am surrounded by the results all day, every day, it no longer seems surprising to me that Kundalini Yoga is a science, a technology for healing. There have already been countless studies demonstrating how yoga and meditation have enormous positive effects on people's health and well-being. I look forward to the day when scientists will study in earnest the very real effects that Kundalini Yoga and Meditation have on people's physical bodies.

In addition to its role in depression with the secretion of serotonin, another function that this sixth chakra master gland, the pituitary gland, oversees is the secretion of HGH, or human growth hormone. By using the science of Kundalini Yoga and Meditation, you can stimulate your glands to produce and use all the hormones you need to be healthy.

The decline in production of certain hormones causes many of the problems we associate with aging. Is it any wonder that people who have done Kundalini Yoga and Meditation diligently continue to have a higher degree of strength, flexibility, and mental acuity?

I was particularly impressed by the progress of a very well known pair of centenarians who were in the press a couple of years ago—the remarkable Delaney sisters, who wrote a book entitled *Having Our Say*. In this wonderful book, they talked about their perspective of being black women in America for more than a hundred years. One of the many delightful surprises I had in getting acquainted with their story was the fact that at around the age of sixty-five, these two plucky sisters took up a diligent practice of yoga. At the very age when most people retire, they decided it was time to take up a body/mind/spirit workout. Certainly, the pictures of them doing difficult postures at over one hundred years of age was inspiring to me.

**Studies do bear out the idea that yoga and meditation can slow the effects of aging.**

A study was done with two thousand people who meditated daily. These people showed a uniform superiority over non-meditators in thirteen major health categories and disease conditions. For example, the meditators had eighty percent less heart disease and fifty percent less cancer.

Another study showed that people who had meditated for five years or less had "biological ages" that were about five years younger than their chronological ages. If they had meditated for more than five years, their biological ages were about twelve years younger than their chronological ages. The study doesn't go on to extrapolate these numbers any further, but if the ratio continues at this pace, you could almost imagine that by the time they were over one hundred years of age, biologically the Delaney sisters were probably about the age they had been when they started meditating and doing yoga. To look at the pictures of them doing the yoga, you might say they were even younger.

The pituitary gland, which is located at our third eye point, is our master gland. You will find in the practice of Kundalini Yoga that we have more exercises and meditations geared toward the stimulation of the pituitary gland than almost any other. It isn't because the sixth chakra is "more important" than any other. It is because this chakra has the ability to radiate health to all our other chakras by means of the healthy function of the pituitary gland.

**The pituitary gland regulates the entire body, and the intuition guides our whole life. We just need to activate both.**

**"It is very important that we work to develop our intuitive power (which comes through meditation), for without intuition, we have doubt, which in turn creates duality and leads us into crises in our lives."**

**—Yogi Bhajan**

In my years of teaching, people often have described life-altering choices they have made on the "flash of intuition." When people tell me happy stories about their life, their work, their loves, these are often accompanied by the phrase "I just knew it was what I was supposed to do."

**"Intuition can only be developed by developing your own meditation. And that means time. We need time to develop our own meditation."**

**—Yogi Bhajan**

A student told me a very charming story recently about receiving just this type of intuitive flash. A longtime student of Kundalini Yoga, she is a recovering alcoholic who has also done a lot of therapy. She is successful in her chosen field and happily sober, but she longs to make a romantic connection and eventually to have children.

She has dated a number of men who seemed "good on paper," but ultimately were not the sort of people with whom she could have a real life partnership. Too often, they were the type who were very needy, but when she needed emotional support they were nowhere to be found. They clearly felt that it was her job to nurture and guide them, and that it wasn't up to them to do the same for her,

She was dating yet another man who seemed to have all the right qualifications. He was a successful lawyer and was kind and intelligent. Even so, she never felt truly close to him. Still, she continued to date him.

Around this same time, she struck up a friendship with a man from work. This man was funny and very supportive of her career. They began to spend time together outside of the office, sometimes going to movies or out to eat, but just as friendly colleagues, as work buddies.

This student was out to a movie with the lawyer. She did not like the movie and felt restless the whole evening. Suddenly, she had an overwhelming desire to call the man who was her friend from work and tell him about the awful movie she had just seen. She began to get really uncomfortable and impatient, trying to rush the date along so it wouldn't be too late to call her friend when she got home. All of a sudden it hit her. She didn't want to call him just to tell him about a bad movie. The reason she wanted to call was that she was falling in love with this man from work. Her intuition kept bugging her until she realized the true nature of her feelings.

She ended the relationship with the man she was seeing and began dating the man from work. They are ecstatically happy together. Although she doesn't know what the future holds, she tells me he is the first man she has dated in years with whom she feels she could grow old. They are now engaged to be married. She is grateful she listened to her intuition instead of her logic.

"Go inside and listen to your inner voice.
Every question has an answer.
Look deeper and listen to that quiet voice."

—Yogi Bhajan

The flash of intuition is the voice of God. Often it comes in subtle ways, and we don't recognize the message. Luckily, the message almost always comes again and again until we are finally ready to heed it.

There is no doubt in my mind, one of the best ways to learn to listen to your own intuition is through a consistent practice of yoga, meditation, and prayer.

My intuition has always been strong, but during the last thirty years, through the practice of Kundalini Yoga and Meditation, I am astonished at myself. I use my intuition on a daily basis, particularly in my teaching.

You will come to accept your ability to use intuition as a tool in your life as easily as you accept the ability to walk. You will use intuition to open the door to the guidance of your higher power as easily as you use your hand to open the door to your house at the end of a long day. It will become second nature to you.

When I think about intuition, and how it is God's way of speaking to us directly, I am always reminded of an old joke that I love. There was a great flood, and a man was stranded on top of the roof of his house. He was not worried because he knew God would save him.

So he sat huddled on his roof, when along came a family in a rowboat. They shouted out to him. "Hey, you there on the roof, our rowboat is crowded, but we will make room for you if you want to get in!" The man replied, "No, you can go on, God is going to save me." The people in the rowboat tried to convince him, but the man adamantly refused to get in the boat. Eventually, they rowed away.

After a long time, a search-and-rescue powerboat arrived. The water had risen higher, and the man was now perched on the very top of his roof. The rescuers in the powerboat threw the man a life preserver and told him to swim to them. They yelled to him that they would grab him with their hook and save him from the swiftly moving water. Again the man refused, because he felt God would save him.

Finally, the man was huddled on his chimney, the water racing past just inches below him. Down from out of the sky swooped a helicopter, and a rope ladder was lowered to him. A voice boomed out over an address system, telling the poor man to climb aboard, since this was his last chance for rescue. Still the man refused, waiting for God to save him. At the last moment the helicopter finally flew away, and not long after that the man was swept away by the rushing water and drowned.

When he got to heaven he asked God, "How could you have abandoned me like that? I believed you would rescue me and here I am, dead. Why?" And God replied, "I sent you two boats and a helicopter. What more did you want?"

**Intuition is being open to God's reply, in whatever form it comes.**

## Sixth Chakra Exercises
## Finding Subtlety

1.    Sit on the floor on your heels.
2.    Roll the eyes up to the third eye point. Begin inhaling "Sat," exhaling "Nam."
3.    Extend the arms straight out to the sides, parallel to the ground.
4.    Close the hands, bending the fingertips to the mounds at the base of the fingers, and lock them there.
5.    Straighten the thumbs.
6.    Begin rotating the hands at the wrists with the thumbs moving from up and back to down and back, maintaining a tight grip of the fingers.

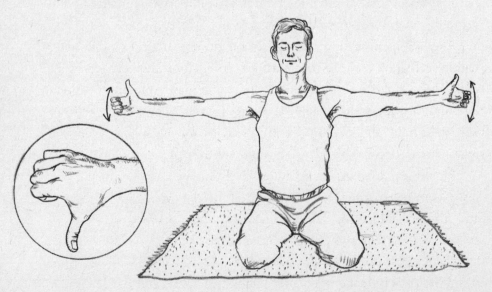

7. Continue rhythmically with heavy powerful breathing through the nose, working up to seven or eight minutes.

*Effects:* This exercise works on the pituitary, breaking through your greatest fears and paranoias. It's worth the challenge—because it *really works*!

### STIMULATING THE MASTER GLAND FOR INCREASED INTUITION AND WISDOM

1. In a sitting position, close your eyes and roll them up to the third eye point.

2. Extend the arms straight out to the sides, parallel to the ground. Place the fingers on the mounds with the thumbs extended straight.

3. Inhale on "Sat" and bring the thumbs toward the shoulders, but not quite touching them.

4. Exhale "Nam" and return to the original position, arms back out, parallel to the ground. Do it powerfully, like a pumping motion. One cycle takes about one second.

5. Continue quickly, with powerful breathing, for two minutes.

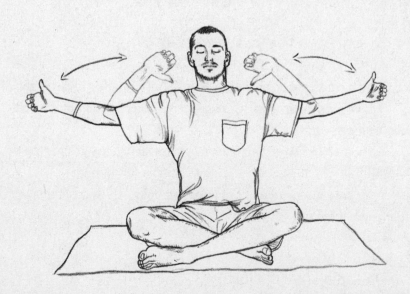

*Effects*: This exercise stimulates the pituitary gland for intuition and clarity. This will then help you to understand the law of cause and effect in your life.

### BOUNTIFUL, BEAUTIFUL, BLISSFUL MEDITATION

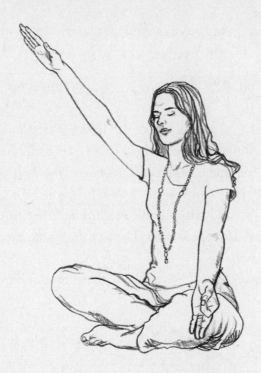

1. Sit in a comfortable, cross-legged position, with the spine straight.

2. Raise your right arm up at a sixty-degree angle in front of the body, the palm facing down.

3. Put your left wrist on your left knee, palm facing up, pressing the tip of the left thumb with the tip of the left index finger (gyan mudra).

4. Keep the eyes focused at the third eye point, as you recite the following mantra out loud:

**I am the Light of my Soul.**
**I am Bountiful, I am Beautiful.**
**I am Bliss. I am, I AM.**

**Say it with conviction, determination, and truth. Speak it to the world, to God and to yourself.**

5.   Continue for three to eleven minutes.

*Effects:* With the mantra "I am, I AM," the ego identity merges into the Universal Identity. This meditation builds self-esteem, self-respect, and self-honoring.

# 7
# The Seventh Chakra

BOUNDLESSNESS

"The seventh center, the Shashara, is the mandala of supreme consciousness and it can be only defined by two words: 'Wahe Guru.'"

—Yogi Bhajan

The human talent of boundlessness is located in the seventh, or as it's sometimes called, the crown, chakra, or "tenth gate," encompassing most of the brain. Traditionally, this chakra is said to rule not only the brain itself, but all the major systems of the body, including the nervous system, the skeletal system, and the circulatory system.

The color that is traditionally associated with this chakra is violet or purple, the color that is last on the light spectrum, the color we see at the top of the rainbow. Purple has often been called a royal color, and boundlessness is certainly a royal talent.

"If the Kundalini energy doesn't spiral into and open the tenth gate, man cannot perceive, experience, or enjoy Infinity."
—Yogi Bhajan

Boundlessness encompasses our ability to connect with the universal consciousness, the Creator, our higher power, or God. In every world religion, there is a term for this vastness of spirit. I choose to refer to it as "boundlessness," because this is a word that evokes the majesty of this spiritual connection, and yet is not evocative of any one religious path.

Martin Luther King, Gandhi, Mother Teresa are all people who possess boundlessness in abundance. They are the true royalty of this world. They changed the course of nations with their human talent of boundlessness.

Each of the human talents is valuable, and none "better" than any other. Most people tend to have strengths and weaknesses within the system. Some people are more naturally gifted with one of the talents than others. I have always felt especially connected to the talent of boundlessness.

I love the expression the "leap of faith." I am physically adventurous and have always felt attracted to the bold image of leaping into what seems like the unknown, but what is in fact the strong comforting arms of a loving God who will carry me and comfort me. The ability to make that boundless leap of faith is located in the seventh chakra, at the very top of our human body, which is our earthly home.

The seventh chakra also houses the pineal gland. For many years, Western medicine was mystified by this gland; and not so long ago, there were still physicians who claimed that it was a "dead gland" that had no function. In recent years, science has discovered that this is the gland that produces melatonin, which is a key component in healthy sleep functions. In his book *Brain Longevity*, which I highly recommend, my friend Dr. Dharma Singh Khalsa also notes that melatonin is an extremely powerful antioxidant and helps prevent free-radical damage from fatty acids, which is a primary cause of aging in our brains.

"Everyone has a sunspot in them called the pineal gland, which keeps a clockwise and counterclockwise rotation. This movement insures that you are either growing more divine or more divided."

—Yogi Bhajan

In having worked with many patients, Dr. Dharma has noted that when he prescribes melatonin, those patients of his who meditate regularly require a far lower dosage, because the meditation they are doing is stimulating the pineal gland to produce more of this miracle compound.

**Meditation increases the longevity of our brains, and medical science certainly seems to be catching up to that belief.**

In all my years of teaching, I have noticed that students who do yoga and meditation regularly seem to have very few sleeping problems, and research continues to be done proving these techniques really do work. Studies have shown that 75 percent of a control group of insomniacs were able to sleep normally when put on a daily program of meditation. Additionally, 34 percent of people with chronic pain were able to reduce their medication for pain, and 35 percent of women who were infertile were able to become pregnant. Studies like this confirm what I have seen over decades of doing and teaching yoga and meditation. It can revolutionize your health.

Such major universities as Harvard Medical School have begun to devote time and resources to the examination of these phenomena. There have been important studies recently that quantify the idea that positive and expansive mind-sets can heal. A recent study of 1,931 adults indicated that those who had a spiritual practice of some kind were less likely to have elevated levels of interleukin-6, an immune substance prevalent in people with chronic diseases.

Having a spiritual practice of yoga and meditation, in addition to practicing a formal religion, if you like, will enhance your health.

**Any form of exercise increases blood flow to the brain, but the amazing thing about Kundalini Yoga is these exercises are specifically designed to stimulate all the glands in the endocrine system. In yogic science, the glands are always described as the "guardians of health."**

In the classical chakra system, the seventh chakra is the gateway to God, or enlightenment. For instance, in Kundalini Yoga, the pineal gland itself is the "seat of the soul." When a person dies, his soul exits through the top of his head. This area of the body has always been associated with the element of light, and certainly the image of the halo is featured in religious icons all over the world.

**"When you have a higher motive and you speak with a projection from your halo, you can win the world."**

**—Yogi Bhajan**

Recently, as science has begun to understand the function of the pineal gland more, it has become apparent that the pineal gland itself is stimulated by light. This seems to be why people who suffer from seasonal affective disorder (SAD) are not producing and regulating melatonin properly. The seventh chakra is the chakra that functions on light.

Again and again, people who have had near-death experiences speak of seeing a great white light, and they feel this light is God. A student recently told me of a near-death experience that her father had while undergoing heart bypass surgery.

While he was in surgery, this student's father described meeting a woman who was radiant with light. This woman, who seemed to be "all love," as he described her, gave him the message that it was not yet his time to die. The light-filled woman told him he still had things to do. This made the man nervous, because he was very goal-oriented and wanted to be sure that whatever his task was on earth got completed. What she told him next was very interesting. She said it wasn't the results of what he did that mattered, it was his effort that was important. God wasn't waiting for him to complete a series of accomplishments. The effort was more important than the achieving. This gave the man great comfort, and hearing the story gave me inspiration as well.

That is the very essence of boundlessness. The Creator is not some awful boss who wants a certain output from each of us. We are not merely employees of God.

**I am not a human doing, I am a human being.**

I love the expression "I'm not a human doing, I am a human being." When I used to hear someone say this, I would realize that it was a very profound idea, and then proceed to get on with my busy routine, missing the point entirely. Recently, this little aphorism has started to mean more to me. I realized I was evaluating myself at the end of the day by what I had "accomplished," and I was always falling short.

Fortunately, years of doing meditation and yoga have provided me with the awareness to see when I have begun to trap myself in an unhealthy pattern. I have become aware of my tendency to focus on being a "human doing." Once I see that pattern, I can choose a meditation and yoga set to help me out of that destructive cycle.

## SA-TA-NA-MA MEDITATION

**A great seventh chakra meditation to do when you feel over-whelmed is the Sa-Ta-Na-Ma meditation. It is very simple. It can be done out loud or silently.**

1. Sitting in easy pose, a comfortable, cross-legged position, close your eyes and turn them upward to your third eye point.
2. Place the back of the wrists on the knees, elbows straight.
3. Press firmly the thumbs of both hands to each of the fingertips in the following order: thumb to index, thumb to middle finger, thumb to ring finger, thumb to pinkie.

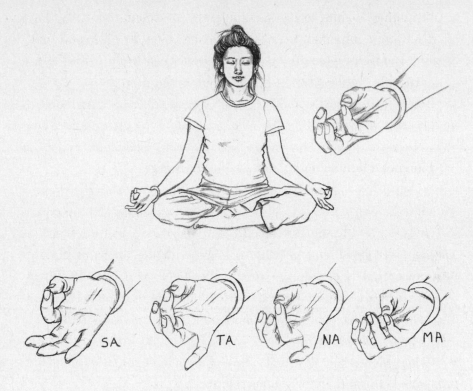

4.  Verbally or mentally chant "Sa-Ta-Na-Ma," one syllable to each finger. Recite in a monotone.

5.  Once finished, begin the next round, starting again with the index finger and ending with the pinkie. Continue.

6.  Do it for seven to eleven minutes.

*Effects:* There is tremendous power in this one little meditation. First of all, let's take a look at the words themselves. They are simply an extended way of saying "Sat Nam," the Sanskrit phrase that means "I am truth." The phrase is extended into four syllables because in yogic tradition these four sounds remind us of the never-ending cycle of life, birth, death, and rebirth. Traditionally, this allows us to remember that everything that is going on in this moment is illusory; in other words, that "this too shall pass." It helps to clear the subconscious of past pain, so that one is then free to experience merging one's consciousness with the Infinite.

This meditation helps remind me that my life has purpose, that life is a cycle, and that God has a plan for me. This plan will begin to make sense if I allow myself to be open to God, if I can begin to live in my sense of boundlessness, and be present right in this moment.

Students really love it and find it helps them on a daily basis. You can do it on the train, while waiting in line, before a big presentation, anytime. I have a student who loves to do this hand meditation under the table when he is in the middle of a stressful meeting.

Traditionally, any meditation that uses a mantra or sound current is called "Naad yoga." The University of Arizona recently did an experiment on the effects of Naad yoga. Researchers used a positron emission tomography (PET) scan to look for changes in the brains of students chanting Naad yoga mantras such as "Sa-Ta-Na-Ma." The PET scan revealed a strong shift in the brain's function as the patients were chanting. The primary activities of the brain were transferred from the left side of the brain to the right front side.

This physical shift is an indication of an enhancement in mood and an increase in alertness to brain researchers.

If you chant the mantra out loud, you receive the additional benefit of stimulating major reflex points on the roof of the mouth. Stimulating areas dense with nerve endings has an effect on overall well-being that is not easy to quantify. Students often refer to it as the "yoga high" they feel after class. Not to be confused with a drug high, this feeling does not have the subsequent crash you get with such substances as drugs, alcohol, or even sugar.

As if all those benefits weren't enough for one meditation to provide, this little gem of a meditation also stimulates meridians that are located in each of the fingertips. As any acupuncturist can tell you, our fingers and toes are hotbeds of activity in the system of meridians. By stimulating them with this strong repetitive pressure, we can aid our self-healing tremendously.

I do understand that not everyone who reads this book believes in God. I wonder if you are thinking this chakra and this chapter may not be of use to you. Let me address this for a moment.

The most important knowingness is the knowingness of yourself. Certainly, even in the secular tradition, most people feel that their "personality" is a function of their brain. If your personality is dysfunctional, we might say you are "out of your mind." So, even if you don't believe in any external force creating you, you certainly must believe in yourself, the fact that you are real, your personality is real, and you exist. Of course, if you don't believe you exist, you are definitely reading the wrong book; it's time to pick up a philosophy book. I think most people I meet are sure they exist.

If the thought of knowing there is a God is difficult for you, try to apply these ideas instead to the knowingness of yourself. Learn how to value and treasure yourself, so that you can go out there and value and treasure other beings. Knowing your own self is knowing God.

Use these techniques to nurture and take care of yourself. My mission with this book is to help as many people as I can to begin to love and cherish themselves—body, mind, and spirit.

The crown chakra, the seventh center, is the seat of the soul—an idea that is prevalent in a number of cultural traditions. Religious images include the halo or the crown. This idea cuts across cultural and religious boundaries throughout the world. In many religious and cultural traditions, the wearing of a hat, a veil, a miter, a yarmulke, or a turban evolved as a way of reminding ourselves of the presence of spirit in our lives. Head coverings seem to occur in almost every world religion. I am a Sikh, and I do wear a turban. For most people, traditional religious garb isn't part of their daily routine.

I see my turban as a wonderful extension of my crown chakra. It serves as a daily reminder of my knowingness of God. The very physical action of winding the fabric around my head is a ritual that allows me to focus on uniting my body, mind, and spirit. As I wrap the cloth around my head, I am taking a physical action, which serves as a reminder that for this day I live in a human body and I need to honor it and care for it.

The winding of fabric around my head at the crown chakra reminds me I also have the gift of a wonderful and complex human brain. As the effect of the turban is to extend the top of my head slightly toward the sky, I am reminded that this body and mind of mine are connected to something higher, a universal Creator, God.

What could be a rather mundane daily ritual, simply covering my head, has the power to be a metaphor reminding me of the things I value. It's not as though I leave my house in the morning, turban perfect, to carry on my day in a complete union of body, mind, and spirit. I can go right into a state of getting impatient at the traffic or worrying about being late.

None of the things that make up my spiritual practice, the way of dressing, my yoga, my meditation, none of these things make me happy every minute. They are tools, reminders, guideposts I can use along the way. Every day of my life I find, as the years go on, more peace and happiness.

**Creating rituals for ourselves can be a very effective way to remind us of the core values that are the foundation of personal belief.**

Take whatever you do and give it meaning. That is the essence of yoga itself. Yoga isn't sitting there and holding your hands over your head for three minutes. Yoga is sitting there and holding your hands over your head for three minutes in order to learn something about yourself. That is why Kundalini Yoga is called the "Yoga of Awareness."

**Yoga allows us to practice knowing ourselves on a physical level.**

I recently had a student join my classes who is paralyzed from the waist down because of an accident. This man's son, a yoga teacher at the center, brings him to class, helps him out of his wheelchair, and settles him onto his mat. Occasionally, the son helps him in moving from sitting to lying down, but for the most part, the man with the injury does the class on his own, doing the best that he can. I see in this man a tremendous amount of faith in himself, and I also see fantastic progress. Within his physical capabilities at this moment, this man is getting stronger to an amazing degree. There are things that are difficult for him to do, as there are for everyone else in the class. His son, a former gymnast, struggles through certain exercises, too.

**Our struggles are our growth opportunities.**

Nothing in any yoga class is perfectly easy for every individual, no matter how athletic or limber. Although this man and his son struggle with different aspects of the class, they both have the ability to learn from doing this work. Yoga allows us to practice having faith in ourselves on a physical level. Father and son both make physical, mental, and spiritual progress through their daily practice of yoga and meditation.

When I say that everyone struggles with different aspects of a yoga class, I mean that only in the most positive way. Our struggles are always our growth opportunities. Usually, when people describe life-altering events from which they learned and grew and progressed, there is some element of commitment and keeping up. What yoga provides is a safe, nurturing environment to allow yourselves to experience struggle, to feel pain, and to learn from it. Each exercise we do can become a metaphor for a larger life experience that we will undoubtedly go through on the "outside." Yoga makes us more flexible, but not just in our bodies. A flexible spine creates a flexible mind.

We come to understand death, our own and others', through this seventh power center. Although all the chakras are involved in mortality, it is the actual death of the brain that is universally accepted as the death of our physical body. This is as true in modern Western medicine as it is in the ancient Eastern belief system. The soul is housed in the pineal gland. When the soul has finally left the body, the brain ceases to function and the body is dead. It is the death of the brain that tells our heart to beat its last beat and our lungs to exhale our last breath.

The body dies, but the soul is undying, unborn, and self-illumined. It has no beginning and no end. It was never born and will never die.

In order for us to cherish each breath we take, we must acknowledge the fact that one day we will surely breathe our last breath.

## EXPELLED BREATH MEDITATION

**In this seventh power center, an easy way to confront our own fear of death and to go beyond that fear to experience the undying existence of our own soul is to practice the technique of held and expelled breath.**

1.    Sit quietly with your hands held palms up in front of you, as though someone were going to pour blessings into your open hands.

2.    Inhale deeply, and hold the breath with your eyes one-tenth open.

3.    Slowly exhale all the air from your lungs.

4.    Once the air is gone, mentally chant "Sat Nam" four times.

5.    Inhale again, slowly exhale, and holding the breath out, chant the mantra five times. Gradually work your way up to reciting slowly the mantra eight times on each exhale.

6.    Continue for at least three minutes.

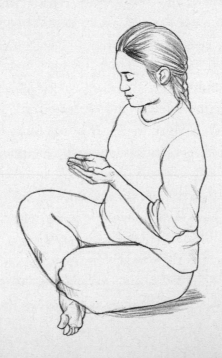

*Effects:* The best time to do this practice is right after you awake in the morning. If you want to do it while you are still lying down with your eyes closed, that's just fine.

Doing this breath meditation can put you through a lot of mental and emotional changes, because it means confronting your natural fear of being in your body, with no breath—which is death.

Any exercise or meditation that causes us to expel all the air from our lungs allows us to be in that place we will ultimately be in when we breathe our last breath. I had a student tell me recently that when we would do these kinds of exercises in class it would cause her to have a mini–anxiety attack. Her heart would race and her palms would sweat just at the thought of contemplating her last breath. As she continued doing this meditation, the fear subsided. Once you lose the fear of dying, you truly begin to live.

This is a very common reaction. Many people might wonder, quite logically, what is the point of this? First of all, the physical action of this exercise eventually gives you greater wind capacity. Most people, even trained athletes, do not learn how to expel all the air from their lungs. People tend to breath shallowly, and they don't fully expel the breath, which means that a reserve of carbon dioxide tends to linger at the bottom of your lungs. If you learn to exhale your breath completely, you will fill your lungs with oxygenated air, allowing you to get more oxygen into your own bloodstream.

Another benefit of this exercise is emotional. By allowing your brain to experience the sensation of being without breath, you begin to eliminate the dread and fear of being in that state. On a visceral level, your being knows that one day you will no longer be able to inhale, and this exercise helps you to confront that fear of dying, so you can make that leap from the finite into Infinity, or boundlessness.

The ancient yogic scriptures say we are allotted a certain number of breaths in our lifetime, and when we have used them up, only then will we move out of our bodies. You will hear stories of yogis who spend their entire lives practicing extremely long, slow, deep breathing techniques, for the sole purpose of extending their years on this earthly plane.

A student told me she had panic attacks doing any expelled breath exercises. Even though she was terrified of doing this exercise, she decided to do it anyway. At first she could keep her lungs empty of air only for a second or two without panicking and inhaling. She would panic and feel she was going to die, even though she had heard me say there is no danger of this happening, because no one has the will to exhale and not inhale again.

She ultimately identified that what she was avoiding in this exercise was her fear and grief at the inevitability of her own mortality. This is, of course, what we all want to avoid facing.

This student, like so many people, was someone who couldn't deal with death, her own or anyone else's. She "couldn't stand hospitals," and when someone was ill, she would always find a reason not to visit. She even avoided going to the hospital to see her first nephew when he was born. This student had allowed herself to live in the illusion that death wasn't something that was going to happen to her or to anybody about whom she cared. By doing this held-breath meditation and experiencing this resistance, she was able to resolve her fears of surrender to a higher power.

**If we don't develop tools that allow us to deal with death in a realistic way that makes sense on a physical level, we will continue to be terrified of it. Yoga can be one of those tools.**

That is why I encourage you to try this expelled breath exercise.

EXERCISE
PULLING THE LOCKS FOR YOUTH
AND REJUVENATION

Another element that you can add to this exercise is a yogic technique called "pulling the locks."

1.　Close your eyes and roll them upwards to your third eye point.

2.　Inhale deeply through your nose, and then forcefully exhale, through the nose, all of the breath from your lungs.

3. Begin to squeeze the muscles of your rectum, navel, and sex organs.

4. Continue inhaling "Sat" and exhaling "Nam" as you pull the locks, for three minutes.

*Effects:* When you contract the three lower centers, it begins a circulation of the spinal fluid up the spine into the brain. This in turn rejuvenates the gray matter, keeping you young, refreshed, and mentally bright!

This technique should not be used by women who are in the first three days of their menstrual cycle, or by women who are pregnant.

Now, going back to our discussion of this student. She began trying the expelled breath exercise only a few seconds at a time. Gradually, during the course of a few months, her terror began to subside. It was remarkable how doing this one particular exercise had, in her words, "a profound effect on my whole life."

During the time she committed to working on this one exercise, she began to make major changes in her life. She confronted her verbally abusive husband, and eventually they got into marital counseling, something he had resisted for many years. Not long after she committed to doing this breathing exercise, a friend who had been a professional mentor to her came down with stage four cancer. What was remarkable was that this student, who previously had been unable to go to a hospital even to see a new baby, visited her dying friend constantly. The more time she spent visiting her friend, the less terrified she became of that feeling of emptiness. She also became less afraid of the hospital and what was going on there. In her daily practice of her breath exercise, the more she was able to leave her lungs empty of air, the less terrified she became of that feeling of emptiness.

As the months wore on, she was even able to be with her friend when she was in dire pain, for the cancer had crept into the woman's bones. During this dark and scary time, this student told me that sometimes, when her friend's morphine needed to be readministered, her friend would literally vibrate with pain, shaking uncontrollably. At those times, this student guided her friend through the same expelled breath exercise she had committed to doing. She embraced her friend and gently told her to inhale. Then they would both exhale completely, sitting in that place of emptiness for a moment, and then inhale again. They would do this together until the nurse would arrive with a new dose of morphine. She helped her friend get through this horrifying pain, one breath at a time.

We were so proud of her, and we talked about the fact that doing this simple breathing exercise had helped her to be able to be fully present for her friend. She seems a changed person, and feels the entire experience of caring for her friend had ultimately been a gift.

She felt privileged to know her friend's soul had gone on another part of its journey. Experiencing her friend's death led this student to a much deeper sense of knowing. She felt no more fear for her friend or for herself. I don't want to leave you with the impression that this period was simple or easy for her; it was one of the most difficult times of her life. Seeing someone who is young and physically vital reduced to a complete invalid was horrifying to her. This wasn't someone older who was dying, who had lived a full life. It was someone only a few years older than my student, a woman in her mid-forties.

Although she felt compassion, the thought of having very little time left was scary for her. She felt selfish for seeing her friend suffering and then thinking of herself. I think we all look at the suffering of another, and imagine how it would be for us. We all go to funerals and imagine our own funeral; it is understandably human nature.

This experience of losing a friend to cancer was very threatening to her. In such circumstances as these, I find that having a physical, spiritual mind/body practice is precisely what allows us to experience what is happening, and not fall apart. What she had to say about guiding a friend through death really sums it up: "I was so grateful to have a yoga practice during that awful time. Because of doing the yoga and meditation, I was able to be fully present in all my sorrow and grief. Now that her dying is over, I find that I experience joy and gratitude in ways I never thought possible. It's like my life was a painting that I only allowed myself to paint in grays and faded pastels, and now I get all the colors—bright, dark, flashy, subdued, all of it!"

**When I think of boundlessness, I do think of that classic image of light, of being enlightened, of going into the light.**

People think that spiritual knowingness involves very heavy, weighty issues. I take almost the opposite approach. When I think of boundlessness, I think of that classic image of light, of being enlightened, of going into the light. In my daily life, I think of it on a more practical level as simply "lightening up." That's why spiritual jokes are great. In the Buddhist tradition, there are stories of people finally reaching a state of enlightenment and being able to do nothing but laugh all day long, as though they had finally gotten the punch line to the ultimate cosmic joke.

Maybe that's why one of my favorite spiritual jokes is a Zen Buddhist joke. What does a Zen Buddhist say when he calls to order a pizza? "Make me one with everything." When the Buddhist pays and asks for his change, the delivery guy replies, "Change comes from within."

I have a remarkable student, a very funny woman who is also a great laugher, who has had what can be called a miraculous healing. This student, a woman in her thirties, came to me because she had severe and crippling rheumatoid arthritis. At the time, she had a four-year-old son. She can pinpoint exactly what made her arthritis flare up so severely. Her mother had become quite ill, and her father had made up his mind that if his wife was going to die, he was going to die shortly thereafter. This student was frustrated because her parents had lost their will to live, and that terrified her. The fact they had lost their desire to go on made her question her own life. She was devastated that she couldn't convince them to embrace life.

At this very time she developed the arthritis, and was forced to take a look at herself, keeping her eyes off her obsession with her parents. That was when she came to me. She was taking drugs for the arthritis. Not very long after trying yoga, she began to realize she could heal herself and get off the drugs. Her dedication to her practice of yoga was very intense. Rarely have I seen someone commit so wholeheartedly to her own healing. After only a few months, she was on the road to recovery.

When this student first appeared in class, she had to wear clunky shoes with braces, and her hands were completely malformed from the arthritis. She was always very nervous, fidgeting with her glasses, and she had a very halting, choppy way of speaking. She is plagued by none of these problems now. Today she is a person who speaks calmly and walks elegantly, and her hands seem perfectly normal.

She ultimately committed to coming to class regularly, and then doing a meditation practice at home. It did not surprise me that as soon as she started to heal herself, her parents began to rally. They are still not in the greatest of health, but they are far more self-sufficient and have a much more optimistic outlook. Her healing from arthritis continued as she kept to her practice of yoga and meditation. She is now completely off the drugs she had to take for her arthritis. What's even more amazing is that in the years that followed, she took Kundalini Yoga teacher training, and now teaches yoga.

Although she was not able to conceive another child, as she had wanted, this student eventually adopted a baby girl from China, something she felt called to do by her intuition. This idea of adopting a Chinese girl came to her when she first started her meditation practice, and the idea just would not go away. Even though she was still struggling with the pain of her arthritis at the time, she made her way to China to pick up her adorable baby girl. Although her daughter is a very high-energy child, she manages just fine running after her, now almost completely pain-free.

As she was becoming a yoga teacher, she got stronger in body and spirit. She experienced God as the Doer, which gave her the foundation of healing. Previously, she had no relationship with God, or with herself.

All her life, she was a frustrated person who had ambitions that she was too frightened to try to pursue. She had always wanted to be coura-geous and athletic, but never was, and then her disease effectively pre-vented her from doing anything physically challenging.

Now she is very strong, and using her body has become her life's work. I believe her soul's longing eventually spoke to her through the cre-ation of this disease. We are constantly being given messages in many forms, which we can choose to listen to or not. This is where yoga and meditation become quite useful — in helping us to tune into those subtle messages.

**The practice of yoga and meditation is all about freeing your body and mind so you can hear the voice of God and the voice of your own soul.**

The truth about our soul lies between all the positive and negative thoughts. The truth lies in this "neutral mind."

When I asked this student about her practice of yoga and meditation, I was surprised to hear her say that although she teaches yoga and loves doing it, in her mind the meditation changed and healed her the most. She sees the physical movement as a way to prepare her mind for medita-tion. Since she has been meditating, she feels as if her human talent of boundlessness has expanded more than she ever thought possible.

For example, when she went to a PTA meeting recently, there was another mother who made some sarcastic remarks about her daughter. In the past, she might have gotten aggressive with this woman or said some-thing sarcastic back to her. Instead, she closed her eyes, focused on her third eye point for only a few seconds, and said a prayer, "Please, God, let me see her the way you see her." She opened her eyes, and the woman looked completely different to her. She could see that the woman, who was overweight and very unhealthy looking, was in pain. She hadn't seen that the woman was suffering until she briefly went into a meditative state and asked for guidance.

**It is in surrendering that we reach out to our higher power, where we receive the broadcasts of the Infinite Intelligence. It is there that we hear the call.**

If the talent of intuition, back at our third eye point, is where we receive the broadcasts of the Infinite Intelligence, it is at the top of the head, through our experience of boundlessnes, that we actually place the call. I once heard someone say the greatest prayer isn't in any scripture or ceremony; the greatest prayer is simply to call out, "Help!"

There are so many ways to pray. In my religion, there are poetic prayers and songs that are part of our tradition as Sikhs. I do believe that the very act of asking for help is all that is required. If you keep asking, the answer will come to you, not always in your time, but in God's time. For most of us, the challenge is that we are not usually willing to ask. We almost have to be desperate before we will call out. As my father always used to say, "There are no atheists in a foxhole."

**A daily practice of meditation makes it easy to keep a deeper relationship with the Infinite.**

I'm able to keep a running monologue going, in the same minute thanking God for the glory of creation and turning around and asking for guidance to find a parking spot. Why not? We don't need to worry about being too much of a bother. God is infinite.

I have had students tell me that they get discouraged, because they feel they have tried to connect with a higher power, but didn't get an answer right away. We live in an instant society and feel the answer to our prayers should be instantaneous, like Pop-Tarts. The connection to a higher power needs to be developed, like love itself. There may be people who can naturally surrender and experience the state of boundlessness, but that's not most of us.

**Expecting to have instant knowingness in God, or in yourself, is like expecting someone to hand you a violin and have you**

**instantly play a sonata. It takes time, but you will play beautifully very soon.**

I love my teacher's saying "Fake it and you will make it." That has a lot of resonance for me. For example, every Sunday, after the Sunday night yoga class at our Golden Bridge Yoga Center, all the students are invited to our home for a dinner that my husband, who is a great chef, prepares. Recently there were twice as many students as there had ever been. We hadn't planned for that many, but there they were. My husband, who is a very practical man, became concerned, sure that there would not be enough food. That's when "fake it till you make it" came into my head. Somehow, even though there were more people, some of the people had brought food, which we never asked them to do. Nevertheless, there was all this extra food, and all the extra people, and there ended up being more than enough food for everyone. People had second helpings, and it was a great dinner, as it always is. I felt as if I were in the story of Jesus, where the loaves of bread and fish manifested.

With dinner, as it is with everything, it's a matter of understanding that if you just show up, everything will fall into place. It's that way with money, too. I have known multimillionaires who are the poorest people I have ever met. They worry constantly about money. I have been privileged to be the guests of people who live so humbly it is impossible for us in the West to imagine, and their homes are filled with an abundance of food, laughter, and love. These people embody the human talent of boundlessness. It is about perception.

A long time ago, I was in India, in Amritsar, the home of the Sikhs at the Golden Temple. I met a family there who invited me and a friend to visit their rustic home and meet their family. We took a motor rickshaw over impossibly bumpy roads. It was a very hot and dusty journey. We arrived at their humble one-room mud home in a small village, with a cow in the front yard and the family—four children, two parents, several grandparents, uncles, and aunts—gathered all around. Their home was tiny but immaculate. The children greeted us with joyous smiles. They served us a plate of cut fruit, and they played Kirtan, or spiritual songs, for us. We were accompanied by an old harmonium and we all used paint cans as a substitute for the traditional Indian tablas, or drums. We sang together, drank tea, ate fruit, and laughed and laughed. The whole experienced is preserved perfectly in my memory, like a polished jewel that I will treasure always.

Boundlessness comes through God's grace. Remember, keep up and you'll be kept up. It's really that simple.

The times in my life when I have felt the most separated from my soul were those when I felt alone and powerless. When I become conscious of my breath, and of the connection the breath gives me with the Infinite, almost instantly that spiritual isolation starts to go away.

When I was addicted to stimulants, I felt very disconnected from my soul. Growing up in an Italian family, we were taught to dunk doughnuts in coffee at a very early age.

When I was in high school I discovered diet pills, which I got from my sister, who had always been considered pudgy by everyone in the family. In the fifties, getting diet pills was easy. Doctors just prescribed them to you with no questions asked. These little pills helped me to study, they kept me from feeling hungry. I didn't consider them a drug, because they came from a doctor. Eventually I was hooked and had to take them every day, although I never increased the dosage. In the back of my mind, I knew about addiction, even though it was never discussed. I went through theater school on them. When I moved to California, I wanted to get my prescriptions filled, but they would not honor an out-of-state prescription. It was at that time that I turned to speed.

After speed, I did other drugs, but I always wanted to be up. I believe it stemmed from a desire to find a connection with a higher, more infinite energy form. I was "Miss Goody Two-shoes." I wanted to make people happy, never to let them see my "down" side.

I finally broke the addiction cycle when I was twenty-seven and entered a Zen Buddhist center, where I lived for a year. But I never gave up caffeine. I never thought of that as a problem—I figured, there is a coffee shop on every corner, it's legal, and the scientific evidence doesn't seem to be conclusive about the effects of caffeine, so why not? Again, I limited myself to only a small amount, which provided me with peace of mind.

It wasn't until very recently, when my lower back really went out, that I decided to take a look at this last addiction. I had to be humble, and tell my students that even a yoga teacher can hurt her back.

I was fifty-seven years old, and I had to ask, "Does this caffeine thing really fit into my life?" I began to feel there was a duality in me. The one part of me did yoga, meditated, tried to live on a subtle plane of existence; and another part of me felt that I needed caffeine to be able to "do the dance," always to be up, happy, the light of the party. The part of me that needed the caffeine was always scared, waiting for its effect to wear off, not sure how I would carry on without it. This dependence on a substance was causing me to feel disconnected from my higher power, from my human talent of boundlessness.

It took a great amount of boundlessness and surrender for me to give up this last addiction. It just wasn't working for me anymore. After the initial difficult period, I now feel happier, whole, free, and grateful to God for allowing me to go into a more subtle realm, free of all substances.

I remember a number of years ago, a student came to my classes who was dying of AIDS, a disease that I generally see as being seventh chakra in origin. He was physically weak and resigned to what he felt was his impending death, but there was no peace in him. He felt abandoned by the religion he was raised in, because they condemned him for being a homosexual. He was frightened and felt very alone, and very angry at God, if in fact there was one.

This student wasn't even sure why he came to yoga class, except that a small voice kept compelling him to "just go," so he did. Being in a community of people who were committed to being healthy felt good to him, so he kept coming back. He had been a weight lifter, but he had never stretched his body very much, and he noticed that he began to get more flexible very quickly. That was a joy to him, because even though his body was ailing, he started to feel the small victories of progress that yoga always seems to provide.

He became a regular student. Around that time his doctors started him on the then-experimental protease inhibitor "cocktail." He had amazing results almost instantly, and today he is a healthy, active man, and feels AIDS is no longer a death sentence for him.

When I asked him about his recovery, he surprised me, because I thought for sure he would attribute his glowing health to the drugs he continues to take to this day. His response was that although the drugs surely saved his life, if he hadn't begun to develop a sense of reliance on himself by doing yoga and meditation, he would never have tried to get into the clinical trial for the medication.

Certainly, if it was only the drugs that had saved him, he wouldn't be the disciplined yoga and meditation student he now is. It is such a delight to see him in class, strong and vital. What is most beautiful about him is the way he smiles. He just seems lit from within. We all are, if we let our light shine.

This idea that our bodies are finite but our spirits are infinite is part of all major religious traditions of the world.

**Our bodies are finite. Our souls are infinite.**

## MEDITATION INTO BOUNDLESSNESS

**A simple way for us to keep in touch with this bigger picture is by using postures that remind us of this relationship between body and spirit.**

1.  Hold your hands over your head and press your palms together flat. Cross the thumbs for extra support.
2.  Breathe long and deeply through your nose with your eyes closed.
3.  Roll your eyes up, not to your third eye point, but even higher, as though you were looking straight out the top of your head.
4.  Continue for three to seven minutes.

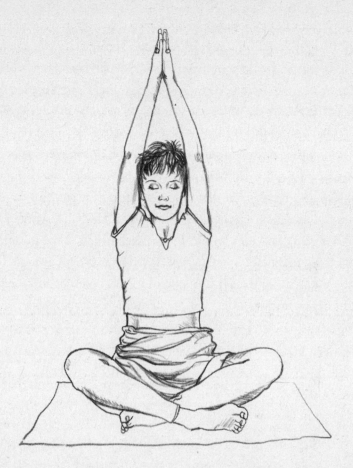

*Effects:* The position of your eyes focuses your energy on your pineal gland. Stimulation of this tiny gland increases the experience of boundlessness, where one feels no beginning and no end, and becomes one with all. After doing this exercise for seven minutes, you will know there is a higher power operating in your life.

This pose is a great one to do after you have been involved in an argument, or any situation that attacks your personal sense of spirituality, your knowingness that there is a higher power at work in your life.

I have a student who works in a very cutthroat business. Her job is to argue and negotiate deals on the phone all day. She is very successful, and tells me that before she enters into a negotiation, she often does this posture for a few minutes at her desk before she picks up the phone. She tells me even just one minute of this posture allows her to see the "bigger picture" of any negotiation she is about to entertain. She tells me it helps her not to get stuck on a certain point, or to allow her ego to become bruised so she loses sight of the overall objective she is trying to achieve in her negotiation.

In her world, this student is perceived as being tough but fair, exactly the intention she is meditating on when she does this pose at her desk. I sometimes wonder what her competitors would think if they saw her, peaceful and relaxed, in that posture before she got on the phone with them. I guess they might very well think, "Hey, if it works for her, it'll work for me." And they would of course be right. Like the martial artist who meditates before breaking a series of boards with a single blow of the hand, she is using the art of meditation to allow her to be effective but fair in her business dealings. She is allowing God in, and recognizing she is not the doer, and that if she just shows up, with a good intention, things will work out as they are supposed to.

**A strong sense of boundlessness means knowing that since things are ultimately supposed to work out, they will.**

This is a truth we can all recognize. It is also a truth that I lose sight of on a daily, sometimes hourly, basis. Fortunately, because I do have a mind/body practice, I find my way back to surrender much more quickly than I used to.

**Imagine the system of chakras as an elevator that moves between the floors of a building, with no floor being more or less important than the others.**

As with an elevator, the problems are sometimes not just on one floor. When a real elevator gets stuck on the sixth floor, chances are likely that the cable may be twisted up on the seventh floor, or someone has jammed a button down on five.

With the elevator of our chakras, if we go in to fix that elevator so that we can have a smooth ride between all our human talents, we will often find that the reason we are having trouble with a certain talent is because we have a block in the talent above or below it.

## SEVEN-WAVE MEDITATION
## AN INNER EXPERIENCE OF THE CHAKRAS

**Sometimes, when I am sitting quietly in the time I set aside for meditation, I like to do a visualization.**

1.    Sit in a comfortable, cross-legged position with your palms flat together in prayer pose at the center of your chest. Close your eyes. Visual-

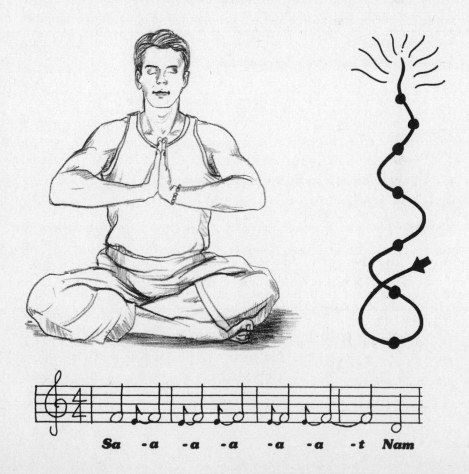

Sa  -a  -a  -a  -a  -a  -t  Nam

ize the various chakras in your body. Take a moment to envision them and feel each one individually.

2.    Beginning at the base of your spine, imagine a wave of light beginning to move from the lower centers to the top of your head, spilling out into your aura.

3.    As you visualize the energy traveling up your spine, chant out loud a long "Sa-a-a-a-a-a-a-at Nam," with one beat of the word "Sa-a-a-a-at" passing through each chakra, energizing it. End with the sound current of "Naam" as it spills out the top of the head into the aura, surrounding your body with light.

4.    Allow the mantra to continue as you visualize each chakra lighting up. Let the energy flow through them.

5.    When it reaches the top of your head, see it bubbling forth like a fountain, energizing the light around your body, and connecting your finite self to the Infinite.

6.    Do this exercise for seven minutes.

*Effects:* This meditation will help to balance out your emotions for the entire day.

**Boundlessness is about letting go of control.**

Full surrender into boundlessness allows the light of existence to shine everywhere, to see everything as part of the painting of our lives. All of the colors have a purpose and a place in the painting. If we stand too close, if we don't allow the light to shine on it, the painting is just a meaningless blur. If we step back to observe, to meditate on the painting of our lives, allow the sunlight of faith to ignite its colors, it is only then that we finally can see the "big picture." The painting that is our life is beautiful and ever-changing, if only we allow ourselves to see it for what it is. It is the true art and creativity of our lives.

## Seventh Chakra Exercises
## Meditation to Realize Your Own Greatness

1.  Sitting with your legs crossed and spine straight, in easy pose, interlace your fingers and place them behind your neck.

2.  Keeping your chin in and chest out, rapidly raise your arms straight up over your head, palms facing down, while the fingers remain interlocked.

3.  Lower them back behind your neck.

4.  Continue, breathing powerfully through your nose, for three minutes.

*Effects:* This exercise works on breaking up the deposits in the shoulders. It also works on the arteries, specifically the main arteries to the brain.

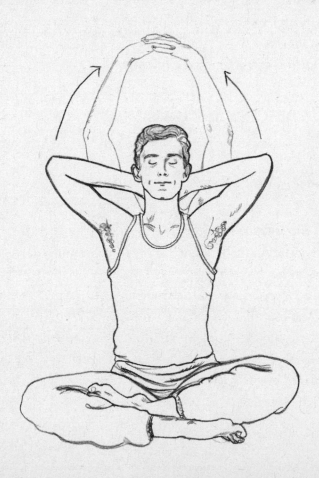

## MIRROR EXERCISE

1.    In easy pose, stretch the arms straight up by your ears with the palms facing each other. The fingers are side by side, with the thumbs separated.

2.    Keep the arms and palms stiff like steel. Begin to move the hands back and forth in opposite directions, six to nine inches out, and then back in.

3.    Move powerfully for four minutes.

*Effects*: This improves the balance in the hemispheres of the brain. If this exercise is done correctly, the whole body will adjust itself.

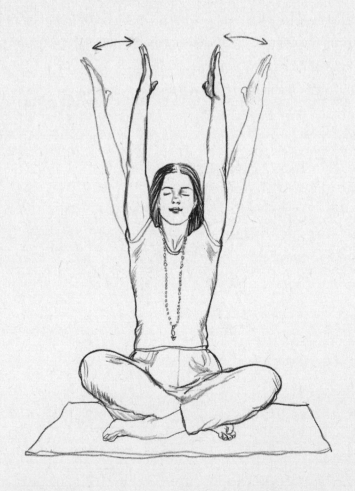

## MEDITATION INTO ECSTASY

1.  In an easy cross-legged position, sit with a straight spine, the hands in *gyan mudra*, back of the wrists resting on the knees, palms up, index fingers curled under the thumbs.

2.  Remain very calm and quiet, concentrating the eyes at the root of the nose (third eye point).

3.  Inhale in three equal parts through the nose. Silently recite the mantra "Sat Nam" on each inhale.

4.  Hold the breath as you turn the head over the right shoulder.

5.  Exhale and turn the head straight. Mentally recite the mantra "Wahe Guru" as you exhale.

6.  Head straight, inhale in three equal parts through the nose, silently reciting "Sat Nam" on each inhalation.

7.  Hold the breath as you turn your head to the left.

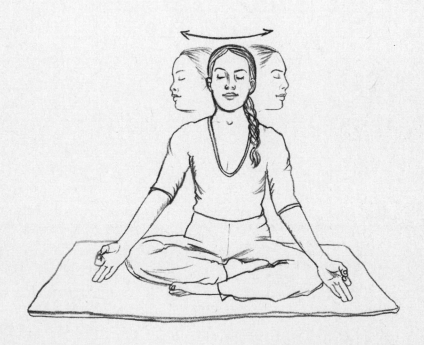

8. Exhale and turn the head back to the center, silently reciting "Wahe Guru."

9. Continue for seven minutes as you project to Infinity.

*Effects:* This entire meditation will lead you to a state of ecstasy and can put a protective shield around you.

# 8
# The Eighth Chakra

RADIANCE

"Everybody is a candle, true. But everybody is not lit."

—Yogi Bhajan

In the Kundalini Yoga view of the chakra system, we see the human form as having an eighth chakra. This chakra is the electromagnetic field that surrounds your entire body.

The eighth chakra, or auric field, extends around the entire physical body, up to nine feet. The quality that emanates from this final chakra is the human talent of radiance.

The color that is associated with this chakra is the color of white, the color we most often attribute to light itself, or the spectrum of light as it descends from the Infinite into the physical realm. Look up at the night sky to see the power of light, which travels millions of light-years to arrive finally at our small part of the cosmos.

**"You can literally wake up another person with your glow. When you are with somebody, that person should feel comfortable."**
**—Yogi Bhajan**

Once again, common phrases in everyday speech reveal that the idea of each person having an electromagnetic field seems to be one we already accept. We often hear people described as having a "magnetic personality." When two people are highly attracted to one another, you can "see the sparks." We tell people not to "hide their light under a bushel."

**"Not to recognize the effect of the aura is the greatest tragedy. Your radiant power has more power to repel negativity than anything your brain can ever think."**
**—Yogi Bhajan**

This human talent of radiance is subtle, but perceptible by others. It is interesting that when people describe a bride on her wedding day, the word used most often is "radiant." I think this is because we are not just describing her physical beauty, but also the beauty of her soul as she joins with another.

**"A true spiritual man is one who lives for Infinity, and whose presence creates peace. If your presence doesn't work, nothing works."**
**–Yogi Bhajan**

It is an acknowledged scientific fact that our bodies are electrical organisms. All of the messages carried on our neural pathways are transmitted electrically. As a result, our bodies have an electromagnetic field that emanates from it.

This eighth chakra is not like our throat or our stomach; it is not something we can tangibly touch. I'd like to help you imagine what this auric field must look like. Imagine, if you will, that you could rise out of your physical body and look down at yourself from the ceiling. Surrounding every part of your body is an oval or shell of energy, shimmering with light.

If all of your chakras are balanced, the surface of this field is smooth. When you are physically, spiritually, or mentally ill, dimples or pockets appear in this energy field, dimming your radiant glow.

**"People lie. Auras never lie."**

**—Yogi Bhajan**

People who are very highly evolved in their psychic abilities will tell you that they can read the past "karmic" scripts written in a person's aura. They can see if a person is going to be sick or is depressed just by viewing the shape and smoothness. They can read if a person is lying or telling the truth just by reading the aura.

### MENTAL EXERCISE ON THE AURA

One can actually increase the brightness, the strength and vitality of the aura just by thinking about it. As an experiment, when you are just sitting around waiting for somebody:

1. Start to meditate on the radiating glow around your body.
2. As you breathe in, imagine you are expanding it.
3. Try adding a new color to your aura.
4. Let your breath be a pranic link to add energy to your aura from the Infinite.
5. Think very high, lofty, and bright thoughts, and experiment to see how you can make your aura expand.

A student once told me of a near-death experience he had. He was electrocuted while working on some wiring. His heart had stopped, and paramedics were called.

This student says he experienced himself rising up out of his body. As he did so, he could see the auric fields of the emergency medical technicians as they tried to resuscitate him. He could see their electromagnetic fields blending and merging as they worked together seamlessly in their efforts to revive him. He was not a person who had ever even considered the idea that people have auras. He had never even given it a thought, but there he was, able to see them as clearly as he could see the arms and legs and other physical attributes of the people below.

**"Not to recognize the effect of the aura is the greatest tragedy."**
—Yogi Bhajan

Eventually this man was revived by the paramedics, and his spirit went back into his body. After this experience he became more of a spiritual seeker, and eventually this led him to study yoga. To this day he remains disappointed that he cannot see people's auras as he did when he left his body. Still, he says it was a beautiful sight, and he felt as he watched the paramedics working on him that he was able to see them for who they really were. He saw the true beauty of their souls, the beauty that is in all of us. He had witnessed their human talent of radiance.

**The eighth chakra is really the culmination of the powers of the other seven.**

If we have begun to integrate all our chakras, and remove the blocks allowing the Kundalini energy to flow freely up and down the spine, this electromagnetic field of ours fully radiates. Once lit, our eighth chakra both protects us from the outside world and projects our true nature back into that world.

**"Your shallowness or greatness of the soul shows up in your aura."**
—Yogi Bhajan

EXERCISE TO INCREASE THE AURIC FIELD

1.　Stand easily on the floor, feet shoulder width apart, with the eyes closed and rolled up to the third eye point.

2.　Inhale very fully and deeply as you sweep your arms to the sky. Let your palms meet briefly.

3.　Exhale powerfully as you sweep your arms down to the sides of your legs as if they were the great wings of a bird.

4.   Then flap them back up again, continuing the movement—inhaling as you reach to the heavens, and exhaling as you bring your arms down to your sides.

5.   Do this exercise for at least three minutes.

6.   Then sit for a minute and assess your aura, feeling its vastness.

*Effects:* Doing this exercise will recharge the eighth chakra electromagnetic field and strengthen your glow. I recommend you do this exercise any time you

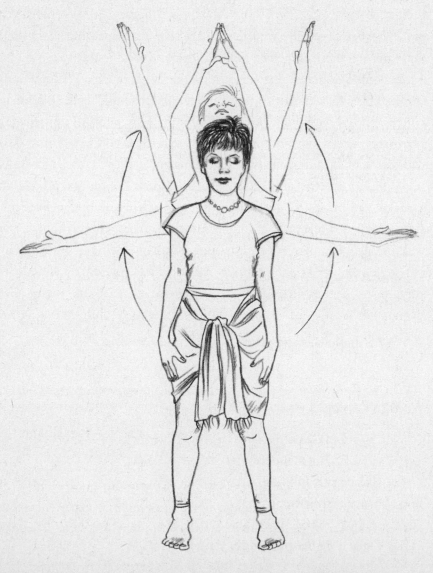

are feeling disconnected, or a little dim. It is a very integrative movement, and it will help you to feel brighter and more whole almost immediately.

The auric field surrounding the body was actually given to the human being as a shield. It functions as a shield of protection. When this chakra is bright and glowing, it is said to give a person a protection from illnesses, to ward off bad luck, and to make a person more attractive to the positive aspects of life. Sometimes you'll come across people who are beautiful in their appearance, but something's missing. Other times you'll meet people who are not typically attractive, but there's just something about them that's making them attractive. It all has to do with their radiance.

A normal human being who is not necessarily doing anything toward spiritual growth will have a three-and-a-half-foot auric field. Inanimate objects tend to have a one-and-a-half-foot aura. If you want immediately to expand the size of your aura, you can wear white cotton clothing. This will give you an immediate six-inch extension.

With the practice of breathing, yoga, and positive mental projection, a person can begin to extend his or her auric field to nine feet on either side, or eighteen feet total. If you are around someone of this caliber, you will feel good just being in that person's company. Being in the company of people who have brighter, more expanded auric fields can actually be very healing and purifying. When two people are speaking, such as in a negotiation setting, for example, the person with the brightest aura will often "win."

"Everybody loves to live off another's power, energy, psyche. Every aura lives through another's aura."

—Yogi Bhajan

People's auras *do* merge. All during the day our auric fields cross those of others. If your auric field is not strong, you may experience yourself "picking up" the emotions of another through your auric field. It is not something to worry about—and it's nothing new, as this has been happening to us our whole lives. You might want to become sensitive to, and aware of, this phenomenon. Take it in a light-hearted way, play with it as you would a game—because your attitude, approach, and thoughts also affect the health and strength of your aura.

People who can see auras will see the color, shape, and size of another's field around her body. The color will change according to her mood. If the person is very angry, she may have a very red aura. If she is spiritually growing and expanding, she may have a bright yellow aura. It is an ever-changing phenomenon.

**Your human talent of radiance is strongest and most vibrant when you are carrying out your soul's mission on earth.**

In his wonderful book, *The Soul's Code*, James Hillman talks about the agreements our soul makes with itself, its guides and its higher power, before it is incarnated into a body here on earth. He believes, as do I, that we come here to learn and accomplish very specific things.

In order to discover whether or not you have heeded your soul's call, you need to examine one thing. Do you feel fulfilled? If you are truly fulfilled in your life, then you are being true to your soul.

If you are fulfilling your soul's destiny, then you are radiant.

## "I Am" Meditation

A very simple meditation you can do when you are feeling unsure of where your life is heading, is to repeat to yourself one easy mantra: "I am, I AM." Say it out loud or simply repeat it mentally, silently. You don't have to say to yourself, "I am powerful" or "I am successful." You merely have to affirm, "I am."

During the first "I am," feel yourself as you are now, encapsulated in your finite body. With the second "I AM," connect through the radiance of your aura to the infinite energy around you. Experience the glow around you expanding out with every repetition.

It's important to remember you are not your job or your race or your income or your spouse or your kids. You are not your face or your body or the car you drive or the clothes you wear. Ultimately, you just are. Keep repeating to yourself, "I am, I AM."

**"The entire human psyche is part of the entire universal electromagnetic field and it is nurtured by that frequency and that touch."**

**—Yogi Bhajan**

No matter what is going on in your life, you are whole, you are complete, you are enough. This electromagnetic field of yours will begin to attract exactly what you need into your life. In truth, it always attracts what you need. It's simply that sometimes what you need is a lesson that will come to you through pain or adversity. Your soul is always in contact with the Creator, even when your human will and mind are not. Your soul knows what you need to continue to grow.

This lifetime is a university, and we are here to learn certain lessons. Your soul needs a body through which to manifest itself on this planet, so that you can use all your human talents to learn the lessons that life on earth has to teach you. The soul itself emanates from the body because, in reality, we are all connected. We do not merely end at our skin, and our soul knows this truth absolutely.

**I am the light of my soul. I am bountiful, I am beautiful, I am bliss. I am, I AM.**

In Kundalini Yoga we sometimes refer to the components of our auric field as the subtle bodies. I love this term, because these subtleties are something we don't normally think about.

We don't have to understand this last energy vortex, because it is the province of our soul. Our soul is wiser than our human mind can ever grasp. Our human talent of radiance is just a glimpse into the vast, infinite splendor that is our soul. We are aware of it in subtle ways that cannot be fully explained. For this I am truly grateful.

### EIGHTH CHAKRA EXERCISES
### EXPAND YOUR ELECTROMAGNETIC FREQUENCY

1.   Sit in an easy pose, with your legs crossed and your spine straight. Extend the arms out to the sides, parallel to the ground, with the palms face-up. Clench the fingers, keeping the entire hand rigid and taut like a claw.

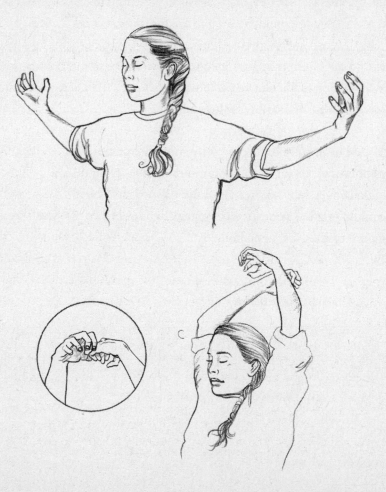

2.   Sweep the arms up over the head, crossing the wrists, then return the arms back out by the sides, parallel to the ground.

3.   Alternately cross your wrists over your head, so the right wrist is in front one time, and then the left wrist is in front the next time. When the right wrist crosses in front, the hands are more above the forehead. And when the left wrist crosses in front, the hands are above the back of the head.

4.   Move powerfully, coordinating the breath so you are breathing one inhale/exhale per each movement.

5.   Continue for nine minutes. Then . . .

6.   Inhale deeply with your arms out to the sides and hold the breath. Extend your tongue out as far as it will go and hold it there for fifteen seconds. Exhale. Repeat this one more time. Then finally . . .

7.   Inhale and hold the tongue out for thirty seconds.

8.   Exhale and relax your hands down into your lap. Sit for a few minutes and sing an inspiring song, or you may choose to just breathe long and deep, listening to the silence while you experience the energy you have built up around you. Continue for three minutes.

*Effects:* This works on the electromagnetic frequency of the brain. The fingers pressurize the areas of the brain related to its functioning. The lymph and nervous systems are tuned up and the powerful breath of fire stimulates the pituitary gland and causes the pineal gland to change the frequency of the radiance of your magnetic field.

## MEDITATION FOR SPIRITUAL AWAKENING

1.   Sit in a comfortable position. The eyes are one-tenth open.

2.   Raise your arms up over the head, interlacing the fingers six inches above the top of the head, palms face-down. Elbows are bent slightly, forming an arc around your head.

3.   Deeply inhale and hold the breath in.

4.   Exhale fully and hold the breath out. Be sure to use long, deep, complete breaths.

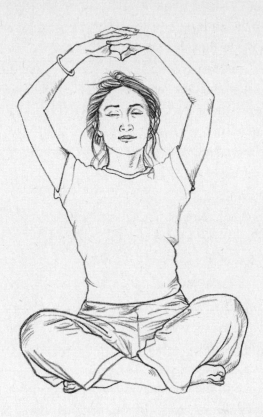

5.  Continue eleven minutes. You can slowly work up to thirty-one minutes.

*Effects:* This meditation is for our mental capacity and creativity. Keep the spine very straight to increase the magnetic field. At first you may experience a little pain in the arms, but go through it and you will feel a deep relaxation. If you honestly do this meditation, you will gain in spiritual stamina.

# 9
# Conclusion

"The science of the chakras was developed so that whatever a person does, he is aware of his various assets. When your chakras are not under your control, your friends are not with you."

—Yogi Bhajan

Our bodies are like complex worlds within worlds. We know where they begin and end, and yet they are vast and full of mysteries we can never understand. No machine has ever been devised by man that is as complex or artful as our own human body.

The ancient system of chakras is simply one way of understanding our own bodies on a metaphorical level. Although we ascribe certain emotions or qualities to these power centers, we know there is a constant flow of subtle interaction going on all the time. When we are frightened, our heart beats faster and we breathe more rapidly; so we may choose to classify fear as the shadow emotion of the heart chakra, as a way of understanding how fear operates in our lives.

Then, at times when fear becomes overwhelming, it can seep into all the chakras. We feel it in the tightening of our throat and the butterflies in our stomach. So you can see, the chakra system is not a concrete system of absolutes.

**Our bodies are mostly water, and we have to acknowledge that just as there is a constant flow within the body, so must there be flow between the chakras, and the human talents we ascribe to them.**

What is useful about this system is the idea that our conscious awareness doesn't just live in our head; it lives in our hearts and our livers and even in our baby toes. If we begin to use our whole body as a kind of conscious road map, we can begin to see how the positive qualities, our eight human talents, can improve our physical, mental, and spiritual health. I pray you will experience Kundalini Yoga and Meditation, providing you with a way of lovingly nurturing your own lives, bringing out the positive aspects of you.

Instead of just realizing you need to let go of anger in order to grow, you now have some very specific physical actions you can take to put that good intention to work.

In this book I have given you only a sample of the richness that Kundalini Yoga and Meditation can bring to your life. I didn't invent it, and every day that I do it, I experience a mixture of awe and gratitude for how much it teaches me about the art of becoming fully human. I am forever grateful to my teacher, Yogi Bhajan, for bringing this miraculous technology to the West, and I am grateful to be able to share it with all of you.

Part of the beauty of yoga and meditation is that we each experience it our own way. What I have learned is that just showing up for the work always seems to bring me exactly the lesson I need on any given day.

I make no claims that the type of yoga I teach is better than any other kind of yoga, or any other kind of exercise, for that matter. I only know it works for me, and that I have seen it work in the lives of thousands of students. That is why the art and science of Kundalini Yoga and Meditation has become the tool I choose to use in my life's mission—to help and uplift others around me.

I have seen people triumph over mental illness, addiction, cancer, infertility, AIDS. I have seen people have dramatic healings, and I assume that countless others have had healing on a more subtle level. Sometimes the things we do in this yoga seem silly on the surface, but I know people wouldn't keep coming back year after year if they were not feeling better because of this practice.

I pray everyone reading this book could come sit in class with us for just one day, but I know this may not be physically possible. Please know that whenever you open this book and take the bold and courageous step of doing one of these techniques, my prayers will be with you.

My greatest dream is for people to realize that they can become the active creators of their own physical health and mental well-being.

I encourage you to use this book in any way that makes sense for you. You can choose each of the eight exercises and meditations that close each chapter. You can simply choose one of the many exercises or meditations woven throughout the book and concentrate on that. Perhaps you will decide to do one of them as a forty-day commitment.

Another way to use this book is to come to it when you are troubled and not sure where the problem is. Hold the book in your hands and say a little prayer, asking God to work through your intuition to give you the guidance you need. Then allow the book to open wherever it will. Open your eyes and see what page you have landed on. Be willing to consider the fact that whatever the book has opened to, that is the message you need to concentrate on right at that moment. Whichever human talent is being discussed, let that be the one you focus on for that day. I do this practice often with any book I find spiritually inspiring, and I never fail to find exactly the answer I am seeking.

**I believe that God has given us human bodies so that we can learn.**

Honor your body. Feed it wholesome food, hydrate it with pure fresh water, lovingly bathe and dress and ornament it. If you stretch and strengthen it, allowing it to have the unlimited nourishment of oxygen that it craves, all the while feeding it the positive encouragement of uplifting thoughts, then this body will serve you faithfully.

**No amount of worldly success or money or knowledge can ever be as valuable as feeling comfortable in your body.**

These tools can give you the most valuable asset in the world, your health, and are available to everyone willing to make the effort. You can choose to be a healthy person, and you can choose to feel at home in your own body. It's not about looking perfect, it's about feeling great.

The stretching and twisting and rocking that you did when you were still in your mother's womb are the very postures and exercises that will sustain your physical body for a long, healthy, flexible life. Not only will your physical health improve, but I guarantee you that your emotional and spiritual health will also increase.

Use some of these tools in your life, and feel the sweetness that occurs when your body begins to function according to the original plan of the Creator. I encourage you with all my heart to then continue incorporating Kundalini Yoga and Meditation into your daily routine. I especially encourage you to take a yoga class of any kind. The benefits of the group energy will only multiply the effect of the work. That is the subtle beauty of the eighth chakra in action—whenever two or more are gathered, the combined energy of the auric fields benefit all who participate. The reasons for this are mysterious to me, and yet I know they are real, because I see the powerful effects of this group energy every day of my life.

If you come to a class I am teaching, you'll discover we always end every session with a little prayer in the form of a song. Even though I hear this song many times a day, I never get tired of singing it or of its message. I particularly love it when the babies of the pregnancy yoga moms come to class and hear us sing this song. They are mesmerized, because they remember hearing it from the dark, warm comfort of their mother's womb.

I will close with the lyrics of this prayer, praying everyone who reads these words will come to find the happiness and healing I know that God wants for them. Thank you for allowing me to be a part of your journey.

> **May the long time sun shine upon you**
> **All love surround you**
> **And the pure light within you**
> **Guide your way on**
> **Guide your way on**
> **Guide your way on**
> **Sat Nam**

# An Overview of the Chakras

The word "chakra" literally means "wheel" and is also referred to as a "lotus." Chakras are energy centers. Except for the eighth chakra, the aura, they correspond to various spots in the physical body, moving from the base of the spinal chord to the top of the head. They are merely used as ways to understand the energy contained within a human frame, and are activated by the Kundalini, the underlying fuel of all spiritual transformation and growth.

The **first chakra** corresponds to the area of the rectum. It relates to the instinctive drive to fulfill one's most primitive needs of safety and survival.

The **second chakra** corresponds to the area of the genitals, where one's focus is on procreation and creativity.

The **third chakra** corresponds to the area around the navel and solar plexus. It is the principal storehouse of energy, which explains why it is considered the seat of power, health, and vitality. Personal growth can be arrested at this center by greed and one's need for personal power.

The first three chakras are known as the lower triangle. They represent, according to the yogis, the level at which the majority of people in the world function. This is the realm of senses and feelings; what one "feels" is considered the truth. Decisions are based on the reality of the moment and a person's base needs, not his higher ideals or values. So an initial goal for the Kundalini Yoga student is to raise his or her energy to the fourth center of consciousness.

The **fourth chakra** or heart center, lies in the area of the sternum and relates to one's capacity to experience and express love and compassion. Here one's consciousness leaps from the inconsistency and insecurity of the realm of feelings to a realm of integrity, wholeness, and stability.

The **fifth chakra** is located in the area of the throat and relates to one's ability to communicate directly. It is the realm of projected Truth.

The **sixth chakra**, also known as the Ajna chakra or third eye point, is located between the eyebrows. It corresponds to the pituitary gland and is related to knowledge, wisdom, and the development of one's intuition.

The **seventh chakra**, also known as the Shashara or the tenth gate, is located at the top of the head, around where the "soft spot" is on a newborn's head. It corresponds to the pineal gland, the master gland of the body, and is related to self-realization and the experience of union with the entire universe. This is the realm of boundlessness, where one can live beyond time, space, and causation.

The **eighth chakra**, also known as the aura, is the energy field surrounding the human being. It is what provides the "hue" or "glow" of a human, and can reflect the general mental and physical health of a person. Traditionally, in other systems, the aura has not always been looked at as a chakra. In Kundalini Yoga we recognize it as a center of consciousness that, once activated, allows a person to easily experience realms beyond our physical bodies!

# Appendix B
# A Gift to You

## KUNDALINI YOGA SET AND MEDITATION FOR OPTIMUM HEALTH

1.   Lying on your back, bend your right knee and bring it across your body to the left side in a cat stretch. Your arms and shoulders remain on the floor. Stretch to the left side and then to the right side, twenty-one times on each side.

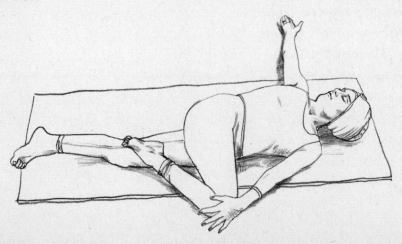

2.    Still lying on your back, lift your left leg to ninety degrees and lower it while lifting your right leg to ninety degrees. Continue alternate leg lifts for one and a half minutes.

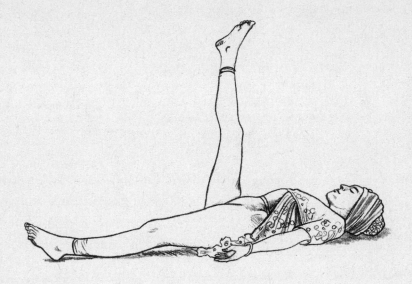

3.    Still lying on your back, lift your arms and legs up to ninety degrees and then lower them and raise them again rapidly for two minutes.

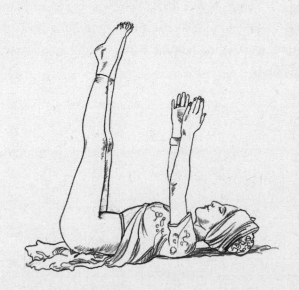

4.   Come onto your stomach. Reach back and grab your left ankle and pull the leg down to touch the left buttock. Then release the left ankle and grab the right ankle and stretch it down to touch the right buttock. Continue alternating the stretch for one minute.

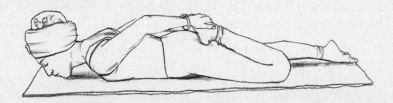

5.   Still on your stomach, grab both ankles and come up into bow pose, stretching your legs, head, and chest up off of the floor. Roll back and forth on your stomach, like a rocking horse. **Extend your tongue out of your mouth** and do breath of fire for one and a half minutes.

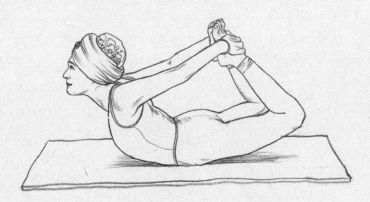

6.   Quickly come onto your back. Begin jumping your whole body all around, up and down, for two minutes.

7.   Come into cobra pose. Lie on your stomach with your chin on the ground and your hands flat under your shoulders. Stretch your head back, push your shoulders and spine up and back, as you extend the arms and straighten the elbows. Begin moving up and down from cobra pose to lying flat on the floor, and then back into cobra. Move fairly rapidly. **Stick your tongue all the way out and breathe through your mouth.** Do fifty-four cobra lifts.

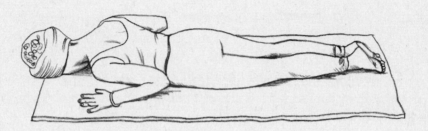

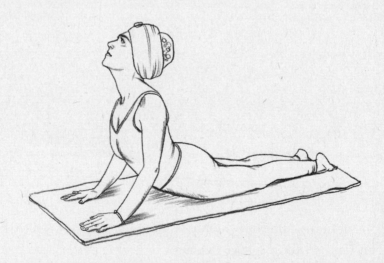

8. Lie on your back, bend your knees and hug them to your chest with your arms. Put your nose between your knees and rock forward and back on your spine for two minutes.

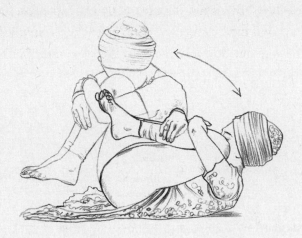

9. Still lying on your back, crisscross your arms and legs rapidly back and forth for two minutes.

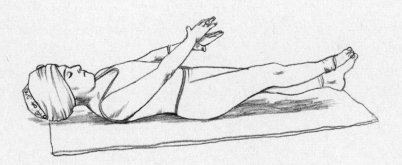

10.  On your back, come into half-wheel pose. To get into this position, bend your knees and take hold of your ankles with your feet on the floor. Arch your spine, resting your shoulders and head on the floor. Hold the position for six and a half minutes. Listen to relaxing meditative music.

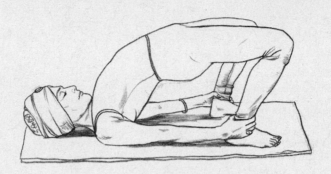

11.  Come onto your stomach, and continue relaxing for another eight minutes.

12.  Jump from your stomach onto your back in one move and relax, pretending to sleep. Listen to relaxing music for eleven minutes.

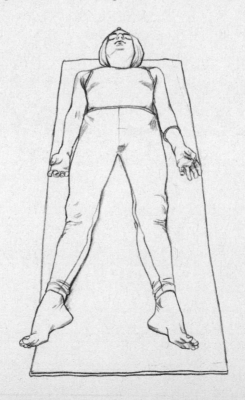

13.   Roll your hands and feet, do cat stretches, and rock on your spine a few times to wake up.

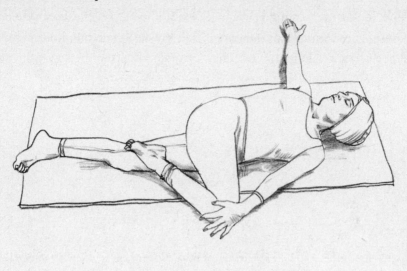

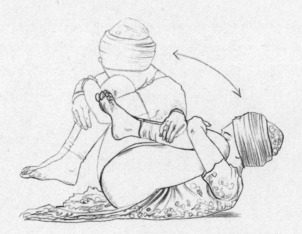

# Meditation

Sit in an easy pose with your eyes closed, looking at the tip of your nose from the inside through closed eyes. Do this for three and a half minutes. After three and a half minutes, change the focus to the third eye, the point of concentration where the eyebrows meet at the top of the nose.

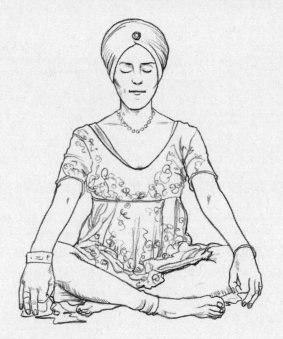

# Resources

## On the Quotes in this Book

My beloved spiritual teacher, Yogi Bhajan, speaks with such poetic innocence that it is my blessing to share him with you through his own words. The many quotes you read in this book are his.

## Additional Points of Interest

If you would like to contact us, or even visit us next time you are in the Los Angeles area, we are located at:

Golden Bridge
5901 W. 3rd Street
Los Angeles, CA 90036
323-936-4172
doyoga@pacbell.net
www.GoldenBridgeYoga.com

Gurmukh Khalsa's website is:

www.gurmukh.com

If you are looking for a Kundalini Yoga teacher in your area, you can find a listing of certified Kundalini Yoga teachers worldwide at the Internet site:

www.Kundaliniyoga.com

For a listing of various activities throughout the year related to the 3HO Foundation, which sponsors events related to Kundalini Yoga and organizes gatherings for our worldwide spiritual family, visit the following website:

www.3HO.org

Many books, tapes, and videos related to Kundalini Yoga can be purchased via:

Golden Temple Enterprises
Box 13, Shady Lane
Espanola, NM 87532
800-829-3970

Ancient Healing Ways
PO Box 130
Espanola, NM 87532
877-753-5351

Cherdi Kala Music
1601 S. Bedford St.
Los Angeles, CA 90035
310-550-6893
www.cherdikala.com